CONSIDERATIONS IN REHABILITATION FACILITY DEVELOPMENT

Publication Number 976
AMERICAN LECTURE SERIES

A Publication in
The BANNERSTONE DIVISION *of*
AMERICAN LECTURES IN SOCIAL AND REHABILITATION PSYCHOLOGY

Editors

RICHARD E. HARDY, Ed. D.
Diplomate in Counseling Psychology (ABPP)
Chairman, Department of Rehabilitation Counseling
Virginia Commonwealth University
Richmond, Virginia

and

JOHN G. CULL, Ph. D.
Director, Regional Counselor Training Program
Department of Rehabilitation Counseling
Virginia Commonwealth University
Fishersville, Virginia

The American Lecture Series in Social and Rehabilitation Psychology offers books which are concerned with man's role in his milieu. Emphasis is placed on how this role can be made more effective in a time of social conflict and a deteriorating physical environment. The books are oriented toward descriptions of what future roles should be and are not concerned exclusively with the delineation and definition of contemporary behavior. Contributors are concerned to a considerable extent with prediction through the use of a functional view of man as opposed to a descriptive, anatomical point of view.

Books in this series are written mainly for the professional practitioner; however, academicians will find them of considerable value in both undergraduate and graduate courses in the helping services.

CONSIDERATIONS IN REHABILITATION FACILITY DEVELOPMENT

JOHN G. CULL

RICHARD E. HARDY

Diplomate in Counseling Psychology (ABPP)

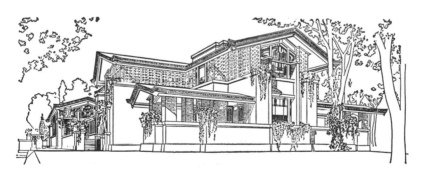

CHARLES C THOMAS · PUBLISHER
Springfield · Illinois · U. S. A.

Published and Distributed Throughout the World by

CHARLES C THOMAS · PUBLISHER

Bannerstone House

301–327 East Lawrence Avenue, Springfield, Illinois, U.S.A.

© *1977, by* CHARLES C THOMAS · PUBLISHER

ISBN 0–398–03347–X

Library of Congress Catalog Card Number: 74–20699

*With THOMAS BOOKS careful attention is given to all details of manufac-
turing and design. It is the Publisher's desire to present books that are
satisfactory as to their physical qualities and artistic possibilities and appropriate for their particular use. THOMAS BOOKS will be true to those laws
of quality that assure a good name and good will.*

Library of Congress Cataloging in Publication Data

Cull, John G
  Considerations in rehabilitation facility development.

  (American lecture series; publication no. 975: A publication in the Bannerstone division of American lectures in social and rehabilitation psychology)
  Includes index.
  1. Rehabilitation centers. 2. Rehabilitation centers—Designs and plans.
I. Hardy, Richard E., joint author. II. Title. [DNLM: 1. Facility design
and construction. 2. Handicapped. 3. Health facility planning. 4. Rehabilitation. HD7256.U5 C967ca] HD7255.C845   362.4   74–20699

ISBN 0–398–03347–1

Printed in the United States of America

K-8

CONTRIBUTORS

C. RAY ASFAHL, Ph.D.: Is Associate Professor of Industrial Engineering at University of Arkansas and has formerly taught at Long Island, Ohio, and Arizona State Universities. He has wide-ranging manufacturing experience both in competitive industry and in rehabilitation facility environments and has served as consultant to firms and guest speaker in major cities throughout the United States. Dr. Asfahl has written publications in the subject areas of project scheduling, rehabilitation facility management, and industrial engineering. With degrees from Oklahoma State, Stanford, and Arizona State Universities, Dr. Asfahl is a Registered Professional Engineer in the State of Ohio.

JOHN G. CULL, Ph.D.: Professor and Director, Regional Counselor Training Program, Department of Rehabilitation Counseling, Virginia Commonwealth University, Fishersville, Virginia; Adjunct Professor of Psychology and Education, School of General Studies, University of Virginia, Charlottesville, Virginia; Technical Consultant, Rehabilitation Services Administration, United States Department of Health, Education and Welfare, Washington, D. C.; Editor, *American Lecture Series in Social and Rehabilitation Psychology*, Charles C Thomas, Publisher; Lecturer, Medical Department, Woodrow Wilson Rehabilitation Center. Formerly, Rehabilitation Counselor, Texas Rehabilitation Commission; Director, Division of Research and Program Development, Virginia State Department of Vocational Rehabilitation. The following are some of the books which Dr. Cull has co-authored and co-edited: *Drug Dependence and Rehabilitation Approaches, Fundamentals of Criminal Behavior and Correctional Systems, Rehabilitation of the Drug Abuser With Delinquent*

v

Behavior, and *Therapeutic Needs of the Family.* Dr. Cull has contributed more than sixty publications to the professional literature in psychology and rehabilitation.

HARVEY C. De JAGER: Received degrees from Calvin College, Grand Rapids, Michigan; South Western Seminary, Fort Worth, Texas and Northern State, Aberdeen, South Dakota. He is certificated by the Sheltered Workshop Program at the University of Wisconsin (Madison) and by the Vocational Guidance and Rehabilitation Services of Cleveland, Ohio. Currently he is Education Director for the Vocational Guidance and Rehabilitation Services in Cleveland. Formerly, Executive Director, Hope Haven School and Work Training Center for the Handicapped, Rock Valley, Iowa; Principal, Dakota Christian High School, New Holland, South Dakota. Mr. De Jager is a member of the Phi Delta Kappa and is listed in the 1970–71 edition, *Personalities* of the West and Midwest and received the 1974 Ohio Rehabilitation Association's Annual *Outstanding Individual Award* for accomplishment on behalf of the disabled. He is quite active in training and consultative activities nationally. Additionally he has published in the area of rehabilitation services.

MICHAEL M. DOLNICK: Chief, Facilities Branch, Division of Service Systems, RSA, Washington, D. C. and Consultant on Sheltered Workshops. Formerly, Program Consultant and Regional Coordinator, National Easter Seal Society for Crippled Children and Adults, Chicago, Illinois. Mr. Dolnick received both his Bachelor's and Master's Degree in Social Sciences and Social Service Administration at the University of Chicago. He is the author of a Landmark Publication in Sheltered Workshops Administration entitled "Contract Procurement Practices of Sheltered Workshops." This is the standard text on this subject. Additionally he has published numerous articles in professional journals in the area of rehabilitation.

ARNOLD G. GANGNES: Received his Bachelor of Architecture at the University of Washington and his Master's in Architecture at the Massachusetts Institute of Technology; he has received the National Council of Architects Registration

Boards Certificate. He is a registered Architect in Washington, Oregon, Montana, California, Alaska and Idaho. Mr. Gangnes is quite active in citizen advocacy work for the handicapped, both locally, nationally and internationally and is a consultant to many states and agencies both in the United States and abroad in the area of facilities for the mentally retarded. He is chairman of the Architectural Planning Committee of the International League of Societies for the Mentally Handicapped and is a Special Consultant to the President's Committee on Mental Retardation.

RICHARD E. HARDY, Ed.D.: Diplomate in counseling psychology (ABPP) Chairman, Department of Rehabilitation Counseling, Virginia Commonwealth University, Richmond, Virginia; Technical Consultant, United States Department of Health, Education and Welfare, Rehabilitation Services Administration, Washington, D. C.; Editor, American Lecture Series in Social and Rehabilitation Psychology, Charles C Thomas, Publisher; and Associate Editor, Journal of Voluntary Action Research. Formerly, Rehabilitation Counselor in Virginia; Rehabilitation Advisor, Rehabilitation Services Administration, United States Department of Health, Education and Welfare, Washington, D. C.; former Chief Psychologist and Supervisor of Professional Training, South Carolina Department of Rehabilitation and member of the South Carolina State Board of Examiners in Psychology. The following are some of the books which Dr. Hardy has co-authored and co-edited: *Drug Dependence and Rehabilitation Approaches, Fundamentals of Criminal Behavior and Correctional Systems, Rehabilitation of the Drug Abuser with Delinquent Behavior,* and *Therapeutic Needs of the Family.* Dr. Hardy has contributed more than sixty publications to the professional literature in psychology and rehabilitation.

ISRAEL KATZ: Has provided technical assistance advisory services to many sheltered workshops through the auspices of the U. S. Department of HEW. Registered as a professional engineer in Massachusetts and New York, he specializes in advising on management problems, production, and industrial engineering aspects of workshop operations. Mr. Katz is also Professor of Mechanical Engineering in the Center for Continuing Education at Northeastern University and Director of its Advanced Engineering Programs. He also served for many years as an engineer and engineering manager at the Advanced Electronics Center of the General Electric Company. Mr. Katz is currently a consultant in materials science to the National Materials Advisory Board of the National Academy of Sciences and is Chairman-Elect of the Continuing Engineering Studies Division of the American Society for Engineering Education.

STANLEY LEVIN, M.S.W. Vice President of Association of Volunteer Bureaus, and Editorial Board member of *Journal of Voluntary Action Research.* Formerly, Director of Volunteers in Rehabilitation Project, Goodwill Industries of America. Served as original Director of the Center for the Study of Voluntarism, School of Social Work and Community Planning, University of Maryland. Authored publications include: *Handbook on Volunteers in Army Community Service, The State of the Art of Volunteering in Rehabilitation Facilities;* twelve handbooks on organizing and administering volunteer programs in rehabilitation facilities, and articles in *Council Woman* and *Volunteer Administration.*

KATHRYN M. LOOMIS: Is a Phi Beta Kappa graduate of Wells College. After graduation she held a variety of jobs including public relations assistant for a division of General Motors; Personnel Manager for Division of Kemper Insurance and currently is Public Relations Coordinator for the Vocational Guidance and Rehabilitation Services, Cleveland, Ohio. She has been active in volunteer work and is currently now on a number of boards of trustees including Beech Brook Children's Home, Cleveland International Program, Benjamin Rose Institute, Cleveland Day Nursery Association.

NATHAN B. NOLAN: Is Director of the Georgia Division of Vocational Rehabilitation. His career with the Georgia Agency began in 1946 and he has served as a counselor, district supervisor, administrator of the Georgia Rehabilitation Center, supervisor of the Rehabilitation Facilities program, and Deputy Director. He is a graduate of Mercer University, Macon, Georgia (A.B. Education) and did graduate work at the University of Georgia and New York University. Offices and appointments held include Past-President of the International Association of Rehabilitation Facilities; Member, Advisory Committee, Woodrow Wilson Rehabilitation Center, Fishersville, Virginia; Consultant to University of Florida, Auburn University, Florida State University, and University of Tennessee in their rehabilitation programs; Chairman, Rehabilitation Facilities Committee, Council of State Administrators of Vocational Rehabilitation, and Member, Steering Committee Vocational Evaluation Project, Vocational Evaluation and Work Adjustment Association.

JAMES E. TRELA, Ph.D.: Assistant Professor Department of Sociology, University of Maryland Baltimore County, Baltimore, Maryland and Research Associate, Vocational Guidance and Rehabilitation Services, Cleveland, Ohio. He received his degrees at American International College, Springfield, Massachusetts and Case Western Reserve University, Cleveland, Ohio. He has done additional post graduate studies at the University of Washington and the University of Southern California at Los Angeles. Dr. Trela has been active in research activities in the behavioral sciences and has contributed numerous publications to the professional literature.

This book is dedicated to two outstanding rehabilitation professionals who have made substantial national contributions to the rehabilitation facility movement:

Olive K. Banister
and
Nathan B. Nolan

SOCIAL AND REHABILITATION PSYCHOLOGY SERIES

The following are selected books which have appeared in the Social and Rehabilitation Psychology Series:

MODIFICATION OF THE BEHAVIOR OF THE MEN-
TALLY ILL
   Richard E. Hardy and John G. Cull
UNDERSTANDING DISABILITY FOR SOCIAL AND
REHABILITATION SERVICES
   John G. Cull and Richard E. Hardy
MODIFICATION OF THE BEHAVIOR OF THE MEN-
TALLY RETARDED
   Richard E. Hardy and John G. Cull
TYPES OF DRUG ABUSERS AND THEIR ABUSES
   John G. Cull and Richard E. Hardy
EDUCATIONAL AND PSYCHOSOCIAL ASPECTS OF
DEAFNESS
   Richard E. Hardy and John G. Cull
BEHAVIOR MODIFICATION IN REHABILITATION SET-
TINGS
   John G. Cull and Richard E. Hardy
VOCATIONAL EVALUATION FOR REHABILITATION
SERVICES
   Richard E. Hardy and John G. Cull
ADJUSTMENT TO WORK
   John G. Cull and Richard E. Hardy
PSYCHOSOCIAL AND VOCATIONAL REHABILITATION
OF YOUTHFUL DELINQUENT
   Richard E. Hardy and John G. Cull

ADMINISTRATIVE TECHNIQUES IN REHABILITATION
FACILITY OPERATIONS
    John G. Cull and Richard E. Hardy
REHABILITATION TECHNIQUES IN SEVERE DISABIL-
ITY
    Richard E. Hardy and John G. Cull
SEVERE DISABILITIES: SOCIAL AND REHABILITATION
APPROACHES
    John G. Cull and Richard E. Hardy
SPECIAL PROBLEMS IN REHABILITATION
    A. Beatrix Cobb
AVOCATIONAL ACTIVITIES FOR THE HANDICAPPED
    Robert P. Overs, Barbara Demarco and Elizabeth O'Connor
MEDICAL AND PSYCHOLOGICAL ASPECTS OF DISA-
BILITY
    A. Beatrix Cobb
ADMINISTRATIVE TECHNIQUES OF REHABILITATION
FACILITY OPERATIONS
    John G. Cull and Richard E. Hardy

PREFACE

A most beneficial trend has been established in rehabilitation. It is the trend toward providing required rehabilitation services to the disabled in their local communities. This trend is beneficial because it enhances the commitment the community has for the rehabilitation of their handicapped persons. Additionally, rehabilitation is more effective if it occurs in the general area in which the client will function vocationally. This obviously is because professional rehabilitation practitioners are more thoroughly aware of the social, cultural, vocational, educational, and economic nuances and idiosyncrosies of a community or geographical area. Thereby the client is provided rehabilitation services with a much higher degree of specificity than if the rehabilitation services are provided in a comprehensive center in a centralized location in the state or if they are provided outside the state.

The purpose of this book is to provide assistance to administrators and communities confronted with the considerations of developing or expanding a rehabilitation facility. Also we feel it will serve as a text for training rehabilitation facility administrators.

We have selected what we feel are key areas of consideration in developing a community rehabilitation facility. There are many other areas which could have been included but to include them would defeat our purpose of highlighting those concerns most pertinent for consideration in developing a viable professionally oriented community resource for handicapped persons.

We are deeply indebted to many outstanding professionals —including the contributors to this book, our colleagues and others. We would like to acknowledge a few who have contributed both directly and indirectly not only to this text but to our thinking and philosophy as well. They include: L. H. Autry, Bob Blase, William Corley, Walt Devins, Tom Fleming and Leon Mennach. Also, we would like to acknowledge our indebtedness to Jean Martin, Joanie Mitchell, Dorothy Powell and Libby Wingfield for their assistance all along the way in developing this text.

John G. Cull

Stuarts Draft, Virginia   Richard E. Hardy

CONTENTS

Contributors.   v
Preface xv
Chapter 1 Architectural Considerations in Rehabilitation
            Facilities Development   3
Chapter 2 Architectural Concerns in Plant Layout . . 14
Chapter 3 Considerations for Development of Contract
            Procurement 37
Chapter 4 Considerations in Developing Psychological
            Services in Rehabilitation Facilities. . . . 53
Chapter 5 Considerations in the Development of a Public
            Relations Program 72
Chapter 6 Concerns in Labor Relations 93
Chapter 7 Considerations for Personnel Training in
            Rehabilitation Facilities 115
Chapter 8 Research Considerations in Rehabilitation
            Facilities 129
Chapter 9 Considerations of State Vocational Rehabilita-
            tion Agency Relationships 148
Chapter 10 Considerations for the Effective Utilization of
            Consultation 162
Chapter 11 Involvement of Volunteers in Rehabilitation
            Facilities 175
Chapter 12 Considerations in the Development of a Place-
            ment Program in Rehabilitation Facilities . 196
Index 217

CONSIDERATIONS IN REHABILITATION FACILITY DEVELOPMENT

CHAPTER 1

ARCHITECTURAL CONSIDERATIONS IN REHABILITATION FACILITIES DEVELOPMENT

ARNOLD G. GANGNES

THE DEFINITION OF "Rehabilitation Facilities" as established for this book, covers a very broad band of services
to the handicapped. Initially, Rehabilitation Facilities are defined as facilities operated for the primary purpose of providing vocational rehabilitation services to handicapped individuals. Specifically, the authors visualize this text to include but
not be limited to the following: Vocational rehabilitation services (i.e. medical, psychological, social and vocational services);
prevocational conditioning or recreational therapy; physical
and operational therapy; speech and hearing therapy; psychological and social services; evaluation of client potential;
vocational training (career oriented); services to the blind; extended employment for those unable to compete in the general labor market.

Such a broad scope encompasses many kinds of environments available to the handicapped, and many as yet un-
created environments for which society may have a need.
Surely no one facility can supply the spaces and appropriate
environments to deal with all of these problems, nor should
it even try. Each segment of service along the path of habilitation or rehabilitation of a handicapped person should reflect
as closely as possible the "norm" of society. This does not mean
that special environments or devices are unnecessary, but
rather that the end result of the process should, as best as

possible, prepare the handicapped person for eventual acceptance into the mainstream of society.

Society today is very conscious of the special needs of the
handicapped. Society is also presently being pressured from
all sides to broaden its understanding, knowledge and acceptance of its handicapped. The traditional attitude of viewing
the handicapped as lesser citizens and their resultant segrega-
tion from society has served to make the job of rehabilitation
much harder. Ideally, one could say that each of the services
described in the first paragraph could and should be served
in existing facilities such as hospitals, clinics, general industry
and the like. Unfortunately, our society neglected to provide
adequately for this "human rights approach." Accordingly, we
now see imperative moves toward the establishment of more
appropriate facilities.

One should not generalize on a facility or complex either to
be providing services of all kinds, or on services to all kinds
of people. The blind, mentally retarded, cerebral palsied,
physically handicapped, deaf, aged and otherwise handicapped have many needs in common, but also many specific
needs. To provide services to all in a building may not be
proper program-wise, and can result in economic bankruptcy.
For example: To provide a toilet, tub, shower, sink or basin in
a building to serve each wheelchair handicapped is wasteful
and unnecessary if the ratio of ambulatory to non-ambulatory
is high. One need only provide a reasonable number, properly
placed so as not to deny the non-ambulatory the right to use
the majority of spaces within a building. It may not always be
practicable to provide total availability.

Perhaps one of our greatest achievements has been our
recognition of the human rights of the handicapped and our
acceptance of them as equals. Perhaps it is being overly positive, but one needs to be able to create from a deep understanding and compassion for the handicapped. Today we are
trying to care for, respect and appreciate the handicapped in
a way that has never happened before. In addition, public
awareness, acceptance and willingness to participate is taking
place. This suggests that new kinds of environmental experi-

ences and solutions are necessary if the trend is to go forward. This new approach to the handicapped requires to some degree a new approach in the design of coordinated services to the handicapped. It makes new and different demands on the architect, requiring a more detailed understanding of the needs of the people concerned. It demands an understanding of the unexplored potential of the handicapped. It demands more than cliches and well-studied assemblies of rooms. It demands a new dedication on behalf of the programmer, planner, and designer to provide the kind of stimulus in planning which results in the non-mobile becoming mobile; the retarded becoming useful and productive; the blind independent, and all enjoying a fuller, richer life.

Too often in the past and even regrettably today, buildings which must be designed for public or governmental agencies, have the responsibility for their programming and design placed in the hands of a few people, sometimes understanding, sometimes not understanding, but without the vision or dedication to really spend the time and effort to produce outstanding facilities. In addition, a factor most generally not considered is the factor of the combination of time lag together with change of method and/or cadre. So many times, buildings conceived by one group end up being occupied by a new set of occupants who may or may not understand or accept the concepts on which the design was based. The results of course, can vary from misused or nonused rooms all the way to dissatisfied and disgruntled staff who can find nothing but fault. Such circumstances must be avoided if at all possible, in the best interests of achieving success in the rehabilitation process within our available budgets. There are ways to overcome these hazards in a reasonable manner, provided that the planners and designers never lose sight of the ultimate objectives.

Perhaps the two foremost and important phases of new facility development are: the written detailed delineation of the program and the selection of the design team members. Of course, prior to this stage, the rationale of what to build has been established after the careful assessment of existing community resources and facilities; after justification of need based on persons to be served, and after appropriate community priorities have been set. Often, the research necessary to establish these facts, can result in a change in direction and priority.

The "team," a comfortable word used to describe the relationship of working members of the Owner's staff and working members of the planning staff, can and should consist of a broad cross section of those who will function within the facility and those who will design and produce it. One cannot have too much input. The judicious and careful handling of ideas, be they from the janitor, the director, the multiply handicapped trainee, the teacher or the shop sub-supervisor, is the responsibility and objective of the architect-engineer part of the team. To "rap" or have basic dialog with those who will make the program go, and with those for whose benefit it is created, is mandatory. The personal feeling of being a contributor to the design process instills a pride of ownership which can become infectious. Conversely, the results can be disastrous. Involvement at an early stage of the project, *of all the "team" members,* is a "must." Too often the general written program thesis is prepared prior to consultation with those mentioned above, and thrust at the architect in the hope that he will produce an acceptable plant for it. The experiences of virtually all practitioners will show that outstanding, good, or even satisfactory buildings rarely result from this approach. Early, indepth understanding of the rationale of the project, of its role in the habilitation process, of the persons who will be served by it and the attitudes and aspirations of the staff are invaluable to the dedicated designer. Conversely, the opportunity to "rap" and have dialog in depth both philosophically and practicably with the architect, will instill confidence in the program members of the team, and an understanding of the technical limitations and compromise options which usually accompany new projects.

Selection of an architect can be done in several ways. Knowledge of a person's professional background or the number of completed projects is not enough. Sometimes the largest, most prolific firms have a relative insensitivity to new concepts.

Often the designer is too dominant in the "team" and follows previous patterns of former projects. Often, younger architects have more open minds; however, the gap between whether a building is aesthetically a prize winner or functionally a prize winner is often a wide one. Architects with a known history of involvement with programs for the handicapped usually are preferable to those without. Understanding and compassion are great assets. Architects with good or outstanding "track records"—by that I mean with a reputation for good, functional, error-free, practicable buildings—are preferable. Architects who have the above strong points and who produce creative, aesthetically pleasing buildings within the available budget limitations offer the most hope for an outstanding project. Selection can be made by inviting prime candidates for interview by the client. Elimination can be governed by a point system resulting from interview. In addition, letters of comment from former clients may be solicited, and completed projects may be visited. Inasmuch as most architectural firms are members of one or another professional society and are governed by a local or state fee schedule, most will not compete with others on the basis of fee (AIA members *may not*), and most will not give free service. One can expect a reduced quality and quantity of service if the fee quoted is less than the local standard.

One important problem often approached casually at the conceptual phase is that of budget. Too often the establishment of a budget comes about on short notice or without adequate professional guidance. This applies not only to square footage necessary to accomplish the objectives, but adequate dollars to build it with. Adequate dollars at the inception of a project are hardly adequate when the time comes to build. The design process can take months, even years, to complete. Construction bidding is based on the labor and materials market which will be in force during the period of construction (which can take months or years). Consequently, available dollars in one year must be supplemented with the factor of cost escalation (as much as 3/4% to 2% per month, depending on locale) or reduced parameters for the project. Early professional assistance prior to funding can be invaluable in achieving a reasonable budget.

As alluded to earlier, the design process often involves compromise. To have thoroughly explored all concepts of design and to have arrived at the most acceptable combination available for the money, is an admirable objective. It is wise to understand, be prepared for and adjust to compromises which may be forced by cost, site features, external influences (such as codes, zoning, licensing) and others.

With the selection of the "team" complete and the establishment of the written program underway, the location of the proposed facility becomes a prime concern. Sometimes the site is predetermined—often prior to program conception, often as a "gift horse," sometimes as a political expedient. Whatever the case, the location must be examined with care. Let me suggest a few words which come into the picture: convenience; acceptability; feasibility; stigma; normal; accessibility; environment. And to add a few more, zoning; building restrictions; parking; transit routes; availability to clients; aesthetic acceptability; relationship to ancillary services.

It often pays off to have your architect or someone skilled in diagramming, to gather around a map of the locale and diagram to locate by pins or tags existing programs or services to the handicapped. To go a step further, one can locate on the map or diagram the locations of known clientele, the distances of travel for them, the location of clients whose needs are unmet, the location of existing services of different nature within the community and the availability of them to those who need them. One can also locate areas where contract services for workshops would be best suited, where relationships to the industrial community are most desirable, or—in respect to health-related services, the most advantageous relationships. At the same time this is being done, a look at the types of services available, and their capacities, will often suggest directions not previously thought of. For instance, the creation of a new sheltered work program that extends distances of travel is hardly intelligent. The forced use of a gift site can often do more harm than good. This is what is meant by the word selection in the previous paragraph: i.e.—

Is the facility in the normal mainstream of society? Is it natural there? Is it by nature of its location, stigmatized without programs or public attitudes?
Does the location allow you to pridefully say "We belong here with you normal folks"?
Has the site any zoning or other code impediments which will hinder the orderly development of the program objectives?
Is the site in a sensitive area where buildings, programs and/or clients will be subject to undue harrassment from neighbors?
Is the location logical, easily reachable, adequate in size and nature, in a pleasing neighborhood free from the normal urban pollutants —air, waste, industrial, acoustical or other?

Does the location fit logically into the pattern of community services? Once these questions have been resolved, a review by your architect or engineer can reassure you that costs of construction will not be excessively influenced by site conditions, i.e. irregularity of terrain, drainage problems, soil instability, other restrictions. Don't fall into the trap of building a rehabilitation facility around and into a remodeled—phased out former tuberculosis hospital or Army facility which is prohibitively remote from community resources and/or removes the client from his family and community. Don't let the politics of using existing institutional facilities be imposed on you. It will defeat your most energetic programs and will only serve to further remove the handicapped from the justifiable right to live in the community with their nonhandicapped neighbors.

It is possible that commencement of a new facility can invoke community opposition. This is not unusual, and can be properly handled by seeking community approval or even support by developing good inter-communication with the community and appropriately educating them to the total aspects of the program. Most opposition is based on fear of the unknown, or lack of knowledge of the clients and the program.

Upon reaching this far in this treatise, a few "dos" and "don'ts" occur to me. The most important *"do"* is to fit the environment to the client and the program. *Don't* force the program into compromise by a poorly conceived plant. *Don't* try to do all things in a facility. *Do* what is natural and conventional for nonhandicapped people. Do not further impede progress of the handicapped by placing him in conglomerate facilities. *Don't* allow him to live in the building in which he works. If living-in is necessary to treatment or training, remove it physically as far as possible so as to encourage the need to be mobile, and independent, and able to accept and cope with the normal adversities and risks of life that normal people face. If living-in becomes necessary, limit it to short stay as much as possible and place it in the appropriate residential environment. To do otherwise is to create institutions or mini-institutions. One basic concept that has proven to be unusually successful is the simple concept of suiting the environment to the task at hand. Nonhandicapped persons enjoy the privilege of living in a residential facility complete with carpets and household furnishings and surroundings. We struggle through the elements to our place of work where we are exposed to flourescent lights, the noise of machines and the fellowship of co-workers. We worship in a church, we go to our favorite recreation spot, we shop in the community and otherwise have a rich life. That it is rich is due in large part to contrast in environment, exposure to different conditions and people. To require the handicapped to function in a conglomerate, tied-together facility is to subject him to institutional living with its rigid spaces, materials and environment. In a recent project of our office, we were asked to consider placing many aspects of a program into a multi-storied building. The reason was principally one of land values, needs and priorities. The program called for such things as a diagnostic clinic, treatment clinics for all phases of medical and dental services to the handicapped, facilities for speech therapy, an extensive hearing therapy and diagnosis center, facilities for psychological testing, psychiatric services, special education for children from five through twenty, live-in facilities for Behavioral Research with families and children. We opposed the multi-storied concept on the following basis: The diagnosis-treatment-medically oriented services could best be conducted in the type of environment found generally in the community. Consequently, a medical-office building or neighborhood medical-clinic environment was acceptable. The doctor-patient relationship would be conducive to as normal a relationship as could be expected. The same was not true for special education. Children need ground level space to run and play; they need to feel that "their" school is like those of other kids, special education needs minimal distraction, children need child-oriented scale of structure and minimum of adult confusion. Behavioral interaction in the family setting, away from home suggested a motel or hotel or apartment-style environment. We felt that reactions would be affected if the environment were artificial.

The same rationale is true about all rehabilitation facilities. The more comfortable the client is in his environment, the greater hope for his successful progress.

It has been postulated that facilities for the blind should follow normal types of conventional buildings as closely as possible. This is clearly rational if we expect them to learn independence.

There are, of course, many specific safeguards which can be built into the design and included in the hardware, that are both informative to the blind, and simple to provide. Literature is available from a variety of sources on this subject. So, too, is literature on many different kinds of facilities for the handicapped.

Perhaps a caution or two are in order regarding making buildings accessible to the physically handicapped. The prime guide to date, published by the American Standards Association is Document ASA A117.1. This document initially printed in 1961 deals only generally with some of the problems. It is, unfortunately, inadequate and out of date. New guidelines will be forthcoming through agencies of the federal government. The present standards for HUD are much more thorough and well conceived. Architects should do more than refer to these documents. They should work with people in wheelchairs during design, and if possible, test out plan arrangements to suit local conditions. Standard specification procedures in many cases cannot be used. Not only the ease of accessibility can be enhanced by careful design, but long-term maintenance can effectively be reduced. What many architects fail to adjust to is the need to supplement conventional space with additional space strictly to provide ease of independent movement for the physically handicapped. It is important to know this early in the game.

Of prime importance to administrators and architects is a clear-cut understanding of each others responsibilities. Too often the architect is given incomplete data and left to design a facility which is poorly conceived and not well thought out. The resultant can of course, be a disaster, or at best a set of misunderstandings which color the relationship. Contract documents as published by the American Institute of Architects, together with guidelines on selection of an architect, and simple descriptions of role expectancies for each, can eliminate many problems and smooth the design process. In these times of changing attitudes, philosophies and methods of rehabilitation, designs can change in process. The ultimate goal of course, is a facility which meets current needs and objectives, and has the flexibility to adapt to modifications in concept. Flexibility is an overworked word in design parlance, however, reasonable forethought can allow for future change in program areas.

The types of facilities we are addressing ourselves to, more often than not are funded by more than one source. Often the sources are many—private, foundations, state, local and federal governmental grants, public subscription and the like. Awareness, not only of the availability of these various types of funds, but also the "strings" usually attached to them, is of vital importance. If, for instance, there is a chance for a grant from a particular source at some time, the "team" should be aware of the design features sometimes mandated by these sources. Many times a completed project has difficulty in receiving support funds for its clients because of failure to meet minimum standards of the funding source.

The architectural design process, as you will see from careful examination of contract forms and as you will determine from your architect, involves basically 4 steps. They are referred to chronologically as 1. the schematic design phase; 2. the design development phase; 3. the construction document phase; and 4. the construction phase. A full understanding of each step, its particular objectives and requirements is important. To learn early that major changes must occur in steps 1 and 2 in order that delays and extra charges from the architect be prevented, is important. We have discovered that the simple expedient of having each member of the "team," no matter how insignificant his role—initial the schematic and design development drawings as they concern his part of the program, has produced the most thorough appraisal by the "team" of the total concept. This is good cushioning for both the administrator and architect against those who later might be prompted to say, "I wasn't consulted." Many things are best left to the experience and talent of the architect-design team. To have color selection made by a person skilled in that work is better than giving the job to an overworked social worker or zealous female member of the Board. Selection of furnishings can also be included in this category.

Remember as an administrator and client that the architect must also serve as a policeman of the budget. Careful work with him will reveal a wide choice, usually, of alternatives. It is wise also to retain in the back of your mind, the appropriate course to follow if the construction cost exceeds the budget.

With respect to a facility whose objectives include extended sheltered employment, or extended services of any kind, one must realize that for the handicapped, this becomes not only his "work," but also his "life." Here is where his friends are, here is where his social life begins, here is where he can be comfortable and extend the richness of his life. If this suggests rooms, or spaces, for socializing, for recreation, for comfort or other personal reason—then they should be considered and provided. Having normal and handicapped alike use the same entrances, lunchroom and support facilities is to acknowledge to the handicapped that we wish to treat them as equals. Nothing could be more complimentary.

CHAPTER 2

ARCHITECTURAL CONCERNS IN PLANT LAYOUT

C. RAY ASFAHL

INTRODUCTION

PLANT LAYOUT DESIGN DECISIONS are often quite literally "cast in concrete" at an early stage in the development of a rehabilitation facility. The effect of such decisions are felt throughout the lifetime of the building. In the press of early decisions in the life of a rehabilitation facility it is easy to underestimate the importance of a good facility layout.

Evidence of the lack of emphasis upon plant layout design factors is the eagerness shown by rehabilitation facility boards to accept donated or low-rent buildings. A dollar savings in building rent is so tangible and visible that it often becomes the overriding factor in a facility building or layout decision. But the not-so-visible costs of material handling, utilities, personnel time, workplace safety, equipment location infeasibilities, and manufacturing inefficiencies can quickly become dominant after it is too late to change the facility design. Once these intangible costs are considered, a basis for plant layout decision making exists.

The very nature and purpose of rehabilitation facility development seems to be in conflict with effective plant layout decision making. This is best seen in a comparison of the planning processes for the development of a conventional manufacturing concern versus the development of a rehabilitation facility, shown in Figure 2–1. The development processes for both types of facilities are oversimplified in the figure, and sequence varies from that shown in particular instances. However, it is usually true that from an efficient plant layout stand-

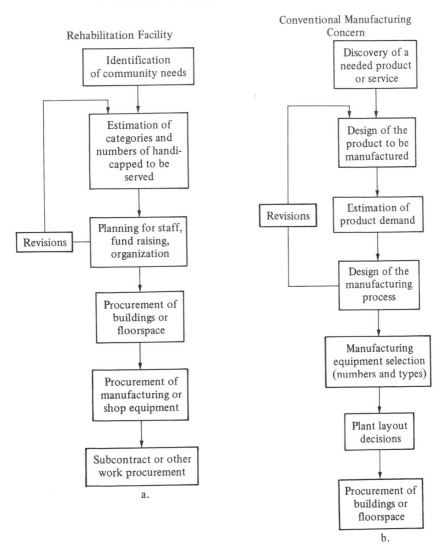

Figure 2–1 Facility development process.

point rehabilitation facility development puts the plant layout "cart" before the product and process design "horse." Sometimes even the building selection is made for a rehabilitation manufacturing facility before it is decided what type of products the facility will manufacture.

To gain an assessment of the competitive environment in which a rehabilitation facility is to operate, one should consider the position of a parallel competitor. How effectively could a new firm expect to compete with a firm such as Levi-Strauss in clothing manufacture, if the firm were planned, developed, and laid out for the process of refurbishing donated salvaged goods? Or consider the position of a conventional firm which had already acquired a variety of woodworking machines attempting to bid competitively for a light assembly subcontract. Such a consideration brings into focus the need for product identification and development and perhaps even contract procurement prior to the plant layout phase. These subjects are dealt with in detail elsewhere in this text.

It is recognized that it may be difficult or even impossible to develop, design, and lay out a rehabilitation facility in the same manner as one would develop a conventional factory. Even though it may seem ridiculous in some cases to select a product or process prior to plant layout of the rehabilitation facility, it is advisable to recognize the importance of this sequence at the outset. It just may be that given some thought the rehabilitation facility might be designed to fill a particular production process need. If this can be achieved, the rehabilitation facility can be made much more efficient and can be provided with a firm position in competitive industry providing jobs or training for real jobs for the handicapped. It is toward this ideal that the material of this chapter is directed, particularly the sections immediately following on the subjects of process design, workplace design, and process layout. Even in those facilities where the plant layout can not be designed to fit a predetermined process, some general recommendations are in order and are provided throughout the chapter and especially in the subsections under General Layout Considerations.

PROCESS DESIGN

Once a product or a production goal or aim has been identified for the rehabilitation facility, one is ready to consider the production process. The process will depend upon the design

Figure 2-2 Flow Process Chart symbols.

of the product as well as upon volumes to be produced. In the case of prime manufacturing the production process may suggest design changes causing a loop back in the process as shown in Figure 2.1b. In the case of contract or subcontract processes the product specifications are more rigid, constraining the process to a greater degree. But in either case the process will dictate to a large extent the layout itself, which is best deferred in the planning process to a later step.

An Industrial Engineering tool for process planning which can be applied to rehabilitation facility development is the Flow Process Chart. David B. Porter's definition taken from the *Production Handbook* (1) is:

> . . . a graphic representation of the sequence of all operations, transportations, inspections, delays, and storages occurring during a process or procedure, and includes information considered desirable for analysis such as time required and distance moved.

The flow process chart employs symbols for convenient representation of each type of activity in the process. The symbol scheme varies, but a popular one is as shown in Figure 2-2.

The flow process chart may be used to analyze the activities of either personnel or material in process. For plant layout planning the material-type chart is the more useful. Flow process charts, whether for personnel or material flow, often ap-

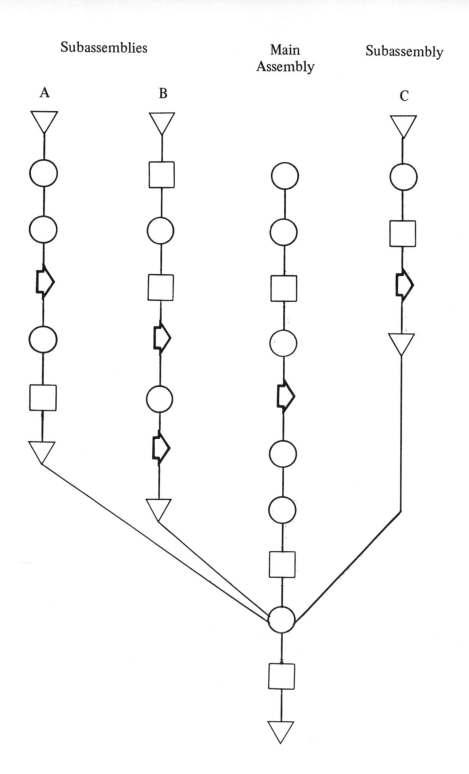

Subassemblies   Main   Subassembly
Assembly

A   B   C

Finished Product

Figure 2–3 Example schematic Flow Process Chart.

pear on preprinted forms. More useful for plant layout, however, is a schematic representation showing merging lines of subassemblies converging upon a single line terminating in completion of the product as shown in Figure 2–3. In a schematic flow process chart space usually does not permit a narrative description for each activity. The chart is intended to give a picture of the general layout of the production sequence and narrative descriptions would obscure the over-all purpose. It is sometimes convenient, however, to identify each activity with a code number and use a key to interpret individual activities.

Once having put together a flow process chart the planner has a clearer understanding of how facilities should be situated and how material will flow through the plant. Although transportation distances and operation times may be omitted from the chart, gross mis-layouts can be avoided by observing the sequence.

WORKPLACE DESIGN

Once a product and process have been identified, the individual workplace must be considered. The plant layout will be affected, especially the seating scheme and the placement of aisles, by the choice of workplace designs.

Workplace design involves a detailed study of individual methods including motion and time study to compare efficiencies of different set ups. Although the detailed techniques of motion and time study are not included in the scope of this book, certain over-all principles affect the workplace design and in turn the over-all plant layout. The Principles of Motion Economy developed by Frank and Lillian Gilbreth have been proven in countless applications in competitive industry and show even more potential when applied to design of a rehabilitation facility where individual limitations of physical movement are often encountered. Nadler (2) states the Principles as follows:

1. The hands should begin and end their activity in a cycle at the same time and should work simultaneously with duplicate parts in opposite and symmetrical directions.

2. The hands should not have idle or hold time, but if necessary, the hands should not have idle or hold time occurring at the same time.
3. The operation method should have the fewest number of therbligs possible.
4. The hands should not do work which can be assigned to other body members through the use of jigs, vises, etc., as long as the hands have other work to perform.
5. The tools and parts should be pre-positioned in a definite location and so located that the hands travel the least distance and perform the fewest activities.
6. The workplace should be arranged to permit smooth, continuous motions with a natural rhythm.
7. The classification of body members (muscle groupings) used should be kept to the lowest feasible for the work. (Fingers are the lowest, progressing through wrist, elbow, full arm, and body.)
8. The motions of the hands should be arranged to take advantage of body-member momentum created through either previous motions or ballistic activity.
9. The number of eye fixations required in an operation method should be reduced to a minimum. (No eye fixations is the proper goal.)
10. The work pattern should be performed within the workplace areas which are considered normal (i.e. do not require the operator to use the trunk of his body).
11. The workplace height should be arranged to permit the elbows of the operator to be above the table and allow the operator either to stand or sit while performing the work.
12. Handles, foot pedals, tools, etc. should be designed to permit the fewest number of muscle groupings to be used for activating the object.
13. Gravity should be used wherever possible to deliver parts to the operator and to remove or place aside parts.
14. When eye-hand coordination is required for grasping, positioning, assembling, etc. parts in a simultaneous, symmetrical hand pattern, the points at which the simultaneous activity takes place should be as close together as possible.
15. Reduce the total skills and amount of work involved, so that the operation may be made into an automatic or machine operation, if at all possible.

Plant layout for individual workplaces is a somewhat different problem for a rehabilitation facility than for a conventional manufacturing facility. Where semi-ambulant or wheelchair workers or trainees are utilized in the work process, larger

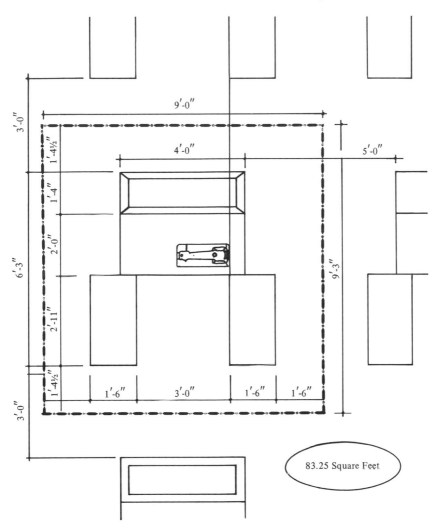

9'-0"

3'-0"

1'-4½"

4'-0"

5'-0"

1'-4"

2'-0"

6'-3"

9'-3"

2'-11"

1'-4½"

1'-6" 3'-0" 1'-6" 1'-6"

3'-0"

83.25 Square Feet

Figure 2–4 Standard sewing machine work station.

spaces have to be allowed for each work station. Figures 2–4 and 2–5 show sewing machine work station layouts recommended by Salmon and Salmon (4) for standard space arrangement and for wheelchair operators respectively. Although both arrangements show use of less than one hundred square feet of floorspace for the entire work station, more floorspace should be allowed when one considers general aisles, storage

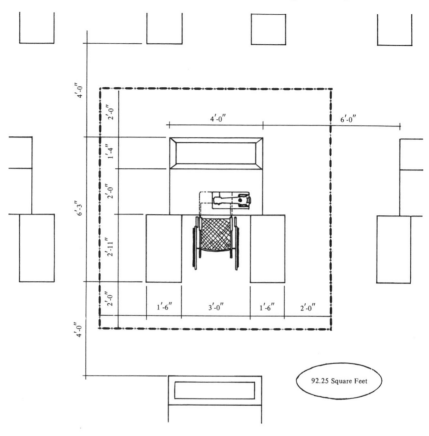

Figure 2–5 Sewing machine work station for wheelchair operator.

space, restrooms, and service facilities. A good average floor-space requirement including support area is generally considered to be approximately 150 square feet per work station.

A tradeoff usually exists between amount of floorspace allocated per work station and efficiency of the individual worker. This can be particularly true of rehabilitation facilities. Consider the four different seating arrangements for a light assembly or manufacturing operation shown in Figure 2–6.

The circular arrangement utilizes least floorspace but is impractical from a service and material handling standpoint. The center area is difficult to reach, and a further problem is the

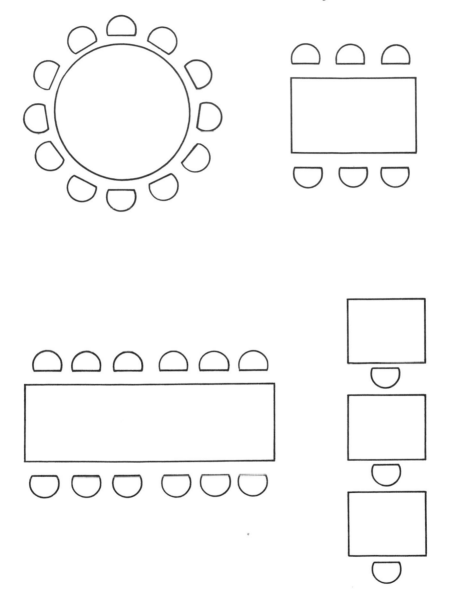

Figure 2–6 Four types of seating arrangements for light assembly operations.

possibility of distraction of workers by their co-workers. This arrangement even leads to horseplay which has been seen to be a more troublesome problem in some rehabilitation facilities than in conventional industry. Flexibility is at a minimum with the circular arrangement if product or process requirements change. On the assets side, the circular arrangement is ideal for some training situations involving instructor interaction with and assistance to trainees.

The table arrangement with workers placed on both sides also utilizes little floorspace but presents a great improvement in service and material handling efficiency over the circular arrangement. Worker distraction level is still high, however, and the arrangement is poor for training purposes.

The one-side-of-the-table approach uses a great deal more floorspace but greatly improves service and material handling efficiency by making each work station available from the back side. The distraction level can be seen to be reduced by noting the fact that no workers face any of their co-workers.

The individual floating work station arrangement requires the largest amount of floorspace of all and true to the inverse relationship between the factors, it promotes the greatest efficiency at the individual work station. The station can be reached for servicing or for material receiving or dispatching from any angle. Workers do not face each other and are laterally separated. The floating work station is most flexible in providing opportunities for design for optimum process efficiency. In assembly operations utilizing a large number of piece parts the floating work station can be supplied with efficient hoppers and feeders for supplying easy to reach parts from all angles utilizing the principles of motion economy.

PROCESS LAYOUT

The foregoing sections have described preliminary procedures for plant layout of a rehabilitation facility designed primarily for the manufacture of a single product. Such plant layouts are called "product layouts." Even when multiple products are produced in the same facility, product layouts can be designed for each, and the entire facility can consist of a number of sub-facilities, or departments. This is especially reasonable when the various products manufactured by the rehabilitation facility are dissimilar and the processes do not employ the same machines or work stations.

An alternative does exist for rehabilitation facilities which are intended to produce a number of products utilizing the same machines or work stations. In the alternative method, called "process layout," the facility functions like a "job shop." The various subprocesses required for each product are not arranged in a line so as to accommodate a single production sequence. Rather the various processes are small departments themselves and each individual product follows a different sequence.

The efficiency of the product layout over the process layout is easily seen in savings of material transportation between work stations. The assembly line nature of product layouts is especially suited to large item manufacture such as mobile homes or automobiles. But even when material transportation is not a predominant factor, the product layout is much simpler to understand and results in ease of production scheduling and control.

The process layout, however, has its advantages and is in predominance in light manufacturing operations which are particularly suitable for rehabilitation facilities. The process layout is much more flexible in that a wide variety of products can proceed through the same machine station.

Machine utilization can be much higher in a process layout than in a product layout. Picture five different products, each requiring a drill press operation. In a product type layout five separate drill presses would likely be needed even though utilization of each might be only a small percentage of full-time use. In a process type layout each unit would be brought to the drill press "department" for processing. It is possible that under such a set-up only one drill press would be required for all five products.

The process layout does not present the balancing problem posed by the assembly line nature of product layouts. In a product layout if a single work station is inoperative due to a machine breakdown or a worker absence, it is possible for the entire production sequence to be disrupted resulting in idle work stations all up and down the line.

The author has seen both process and product type layouts in actual use in rehabilitation facilities visited. Some facilities use an assembly line approach for an important product, or perhaps a bulky product, with the remainder of the facility laid out in process layout fashion. Even in process type layouts it is advisable to consider the process sequence of major products to assist in the selection of general areas for various type processes. A flow process chart, useful for product type layouts, still has application for process layouts in analyzing the movement of materials and production sequences of major products.

GENERAL LAYOUT CONSIDERATIONS

The effective plant layout of a rehabilitation facility is subject to some general considerations, regardless of the product or process for which the facility is designed.

Compressed Air

The very nature of the type of work done in almost any rehabilitation facility is such that the operation would benefit from the use of compressed air at the work station. Provision for compressed air makes possible a wide range of assembly jigs and fixtures to facilitate handling, positioning, and tool operation. In light assembly and manufacturing work air-operated fixtures are most beneficial. Especially in the rehabilitation facility work station is it desirable to design capability for foot or other alternate means of equipment actuation in contrast to the needs of a conventional manufacturing facility which can sometimes get by with such inefficiencies as hand-held piece parts. Compressed air makes many such alternate work station designs possible by providing a very flexible source of power to unusual positions by the simple press of a button or kick of a pedal.

In plant layout planning provision should be made for location of the compressor unit. The unit should be segregated from the production area in either a small room or a separate building outside the main building. The reason for the need for separation is the noise generated by the typical compressor unit. In addition, belts and pulleys associated with air compressors can sometimes represent a safety hazard, especially among handicapped personnel in a rehabilitation facility.

The building or room should not be larger than is necessary to house the equipment. The reason for this recommendation is to prevent the need for entry into the room for reasons other than to tend the equipment itself. Compressor rooms that are too large are sometimes used for general storage, which opens the door to trouble from a safety standpoint. It is wise, however, to allow space for a back-up compressor in case the main compressor malfunctions or is inoperative for preventive maintenance. As a general recommendation, a 7' x 10' space is usually suitable for a compressor room. Optimum size actually would depend upon power and capacity requirements of the system, a consideration too detailed to be considered in this text. Equipment representatives are helpful in this regard.

One word of caution is in order on the subject of compressed air equipment. System pressure is only one design factor of importance. More easily overlooked are factors of power and tank capacity. One rehabilitation facility visited by the author had been furnished compressed air staplers for use in a furniture upholstery operation. On an equipment grant the facility purchased an air compressor of the correct rated pressure for operation of the upholstery stapler. Then after installation, to the dismay of all concerned, it was discovered that the system was of insufficient power to supply the stapler adequately. The operator would actuate the stapler for a few cycles and then be required to stop and wait for the system to build back sufficient pressure to continue the operation. This defeats the entire purpose of use of the compressed air system to promote operator efficiency.

Lighting

Another factor of general application is lighting. The type of operation performed in a rehabilitation facility if often of a bench-type nature, involving long periods of repetition. A rehabilitation facility worker who has one or more handicaps but does possess a good pair of eyes deserves optimum lighting conditions in order to make use of his best capabilities. Further, a person who is partially blind often needs ideal lighting conditions to make performance of his work physically feasible. Recommended lighting levels range from one hundred footcandles or more for extremely difficult and detailed seeing tasks over extended periods of time down to five footcandles for infrequently used storerooms. Certainly a minimum recommended lighting level for table or bench type assembly work in a rehabilitation facility would be no less than forty footcandles. The author has seen many instances of such work in rehabilitation facilities with lighting levels less than twenty footcandles.

The lighting problem can be faced in the facility layout and development period if the rehabilitation facilty planners are aware of special lighting needs at the outset and keep the architect informed. The architect himself can make use of the services of lighting experts who are often available from lighting equipment distributors. In a relayout scheme or in a conversion of previously occupied building to a rehabilitation facility, the facility director or planner is sometimes surprised to learn how much technical assistance to which he has access through his lighting equipment distributor. One, of course, must remember that the lighting equipment distributor is in the business to sell lighting and the rehabilitation facility director or planner should inquire as to levels of foot-candles being provided under the lighting scheme being recommended by the lighting distributor. This is especially true in view of energy shortage conditions which appear to be likely for the remainder of the twentieth century.

Electric Power

Even in plants equipped with compressed air at the work station, readily available electric power is usually required. Consultation with the architect is advisable to assure provision in advance. Continuous systems are usually preferable to individual receptacles due to their flexibility. Individual receptacles mounted from the floor present a shock hazard (in standing water or during mopping) unless raised from floor level, which causes a trip hazard.

Overhead continuous system, "bus bars," are widely used and provide a source of power at any point along the length of the bar or rail. Movement of work stations, plant re-layouts, and multiple outlet needs are easily handled by such an overhead continuous system. A word of warning is in order regarding planning for these systems however. In one rehabilitation facility visited by the author, construction had just been completed on a new facility built with support of a federal construction grant. After construction was complete it was discovered that the overhead bus bars had been installed above the hanging lighting fixtures, causing a great deal of inconvenience to the user.

Safety

A plant layout matter of universal concern is worker safety. Safety slogans, posters, and pep talks are of little value if the rehabilitation facility has been planned and laid out without due regard for safety.

Situations which would be only mildly dangerous or not dangerous at all in the conventional manufacturing setting can become very dangerous in the presence of untrained personnel in a rehabilitation facility. Operating at its best, a rehabilitation facility is training employees to assume good industrial jobs, and the turnover rate is high as skilled personnel move out of the shop and are replaced with new trainees. High turnover of personnel means unfamiliar surroundings and lack of awareness of the hazards peculiar to the facility. At the other end of the spectrum is the situation where a rehabilitation facility is unable to train and place severely handicapped personnel into jobs in competitive industry. Such severely handicapped personnel often remain in the facility as terminal employees, and, though they may become familiar with the surroundings, their particular handicap may contribute to a condition of being careless or accident-prone.

Passage of sweeping federal legislation in 1970 marked a

dramatic change in administration of safety and health in the workplace in the United States. Before 1970, occupational safety and health was largely a matter of good business sense and was desirable in the interest of the general well-being of employees, and indirectly to employers. But with 1970 came the federal government's right to promulgate occupational safety and health standards, enter establishments without warning, write citations, and assess penalties for observed violations. Unsafe conditions which formerly were in the realm of "we've got to get that fixed someday" became subject to possible penalties of up to $1000 per day per violation (3). Coverage applies to both profit and non-profit employer establishments. State agencies and political subdivisions are exempt unless the state's plan is approved by the federal government. Most rehabilitation facilities are not themselves state agencies and are covered regardless of the approval of the particular state's occupational safety and health plan.

Architectural concerns are directly involved in many federal occupational safety and health standards. High on the list of frequently cited standards in the early 1970's was the standard which applies to protection of open-sided floors, platforms, and runways, quoted as follows:

> 29 CFR 1910.23(c) (1) Protection of open-sided floors, platforms, and runways. Every open-sided floor or platform four feet or more above adjacent floor or ground level shall be guarded by a standard railing (or the equivalent as specified in paragraph (e) (3) of this section) on all open sides, except where there is entrance to a ramp, stairway, or fixed ladder. . . .

The seriousness, and accordingly the dollar level of the penalty assessed, for such a violation would no doubt be higher for a rehabilitation facility than for a conventional manufacturing facility of the same size. Once a federal inspector reflects upon the possible injury to a wheel-chair employee, or a nearly blind employee, from exposure to an open-sided floor or platform, it is easy for him to construct a rationale for upgrading the seriousness of the offense. Rehabilitation facility planners and administrators are well aware of the willingness of the U. S. Department of Labor to vigorously enforce violations of labor laws by rehabilitation facilities through experience with the Fair Labor Standards Act. The Occupational Safety and Health Act of 1970, administered chiefly by the U. S. Department of Labor, has already shown its impact upon U. S. industry to be greater than that of the Fair Labor Standards Act. Rehabilitation facility directors would be well-advised to consider the implications of emerging governmental occupational safety and health programs and to plan their facilities accordingly. This is a matter of direct concern for the welfare of the handicapped of our country as well as for the continued existence of the rehabilitation facility itself.

Worker safety hazards due to physical facilities and layout are especially prevalent when the building used is rented or furnished rent free to the rehabilitation facility. When a building is designed for one activity and used for another the possibility for accident often increases as does utilities charges, material handling inefficiencies, and other items mentioned earlier in this chapter. For example, the recent trend to relocate automobile agencies from inner city to suburban areas makes available a large number of buildings for possible acquisition or rental by rehabilitation facilities. The service areas of these buildings are often considered for possible areas for manufacturing or for material storage. When such a building is being considered for acquisition the presence of such items as open service pits and floor trip hazards needs to be remedied and allowed for in the planning phase.

Lack of appropriate machine guarding is a frequent cause of equipment obsolescense as new safety features are invented and regulations to ban older models are promulgated. The facilities planner should be wary of donations to the rehabilitation facility of seemingly good equipment in excellent working order. It is possible for such equipment to not only be inefficient or obsolete from a production standpoint but also to be in violation of federal standards for safety.

Industrial Noise

Industrial noise is a worker environment problem directly affected by architectural and plant layout decisions. Use of

Inaudible, threshold of human hearing	0 decibels
General office work	45 decibels
Noisy restaurant	70 decibels
Point of commencement of hearing pain	130 decibels

Figure 2–7 Sample noise levels.

compressed air operated actuators and positioners can be noisy and perhaps raise the noise level to the legal maximum of ninety decibels average for continuous eight hour exposure. It must be remembered that background noise levels are additive, and the entire summation is what the person hears. For a comparison of noise levels, Figure 2–7 provides approximate noise levels for familiar environments.

Although serious noise problems can be attenuated by personal protective equipment such as earmuffs, the better solution is isolation of the noise source. Particularly noisy processes can be placed into separate rooms with walls of sound absorbing material. Even if the operator of a particularly noisy machine is exposed in a separate room or cubicle for the process, he is protected from background noise exposure, and the noisy process in question is prevented from contributing to the background noise in other parts of the facility.

Aisle Width

Aisle width must provide sufficient safe clearances for passage of mechanical handling equipment if such equipment is used, according to federal safety regulations (29 CFR 1910.22(b) (1)). More specific dimensions for aisle width may be required by state law in some instances, and the planner should be aware of state and local regulations.

Lunchroom Facilities

Provision for lunchroom facilities is of general importance in the rehabilitation facility plant layout decision. Although a lunchroom is not mandatory, it is a highly desirable feature in a rehabilitation facility. The obvious reason is the lack of convenient mobility for large percentages of handicapped personnel. Physical, mental, and emotional handicaps together or taken separately almost always impair the mobility of the individual, making off-facility lunch breaks infeasible for many personnel.

Federal regulations apply to lunchroom facilities at the workplace. Even if food or beverages are brought from home by employees and not dispensed by a central food service, occupational safety and health regulations apply to provisions for facilities for consumption and storage. Neither the food or beverage storage area nor the consumption area is permitted to be located in a toilet room or exposed to a toxic material area. Smooth, corrosion-resistant, easily cleanable or disposable receptacles for disposal of waste food must be provided.

Interior Walls

Erection of interior walls in a rehabilitation facility should be avoided unless necessary to reduce environmental noise. Interior walls represent barriers to the material handling system, increase the need for supervision, and greatly reduce flexibility of the floorspace. Removal of interior walls in a rented or previously occupied building is sometimes impossible due to structural reasons. Non-bearing walls, however, should be candidates for removal from the manufacturing area, especially to accommodate a particular manufacturing process. The author has seen several examples of highly compartmentalized plant layouts for rehabilitation facilities in cases where the facility is housed in a low-rent or furnished building. One such facility was a veritable honeycomb of small rooms which had formerly been used as private offices and had been assumed by a rehabilitation facility for a manufacturing area. Material was being transferred from room to room by means of wheelbarrows. Upon recommendation to remove interior walls, the building landlord was contacted, permission was quickly granted, and wall demolition was begun on the same day. This example shows that a determined rehabilitation facility director can often make needed plant layout changes even in rented buildings. If shown the efficiencies to be gained by the re-layout, the building landlord will likely feel that removal of interior walls to facilitate the new plan will enhance the value of his property.

Loading Docks

Whether a rehabilitation facility is intended to perform salvage and refurbishing operations upon donated household goods or perform industrial subcontracts, a truck loading dock is an important item to specify in a facility plant layout. This point might seem elementary but many rehabilitation facilities throughout the country today operate without the convenience of a loading dock. Such a situation is usually the product of accepting a vacant or low-rent building to get operations of the facility underway. Temporary facilities which evolve into permanent facilities may do so often because plant layout and other inefficiencies prevent the kind of competitive operation which leads to increased volumes of work and subsequent needs for physical plant expansions for the rehabilitation facility.

Parking

An architect preparing layouts for a rehabilitation facility should be advised concerning the motor vehicle parking needs peculiar to a rehabilitation facility. An ordinary factory of comparable size to the planned rehabilitation facility, in terms of numbers of employees, will normally require more automobile parking spaces than will the rehabilitation facility. The reduced level of mobility among handicapped personnel causes a noticeable difference in the number of vehicles driven by personnel to and from the facility. Rehabilitation facilities often employ buses to transport handicapped personnel to and from work each day. The architect should attempt to arrange the parking area so that a bus or van-type vehicle can load and unload occupants preferably without the necessity of backing out of a parking space.

The automobile parking spaces which are provided should be oversize to permit space for loading and unloading of semi-ambulant and wheelchair occupants. Salmon and Salmon recommend eleven-feet-wide spaces for semi-ambulant personnel and twelve-feet-wide spaces for wheelchair personnel compared to the normal nine-feet-wide parking space (4).

Expansion

It is wise at the outset of planning for a rehabilitation facility to allow lot space for expanding the building as may be required in the future. This point was demonstrated in a dramatic way on a consultative visit to a rehabilitation facility. Quite ironically it was just such lack of planning on the part of a firm in the ranks of competitive industry that led to opportunity for a subcontract with the rehabilitation facility. The firm was boxed in by streets on two sides, a railroad on the third, and a cemetery on the fourth. The plant manager had succeeded in many ingenious ways to increase output within a given floorspace but was finally forced to seek sources of subcontract assistance to satisfy production demands. The lesson to be learned is that a little extra investment in land at the outset will frequently be very important to the future of the rehabilitation facility. As new methods of training and orientation for handicapped personnel are devised, needs for floorspace will expand.

Akin to the need for allowing for space for expansion is the need for flexibility in facilities layout. Community needs change, personnel levels change, and industrial subcontracts come and go. To remain efficient and to bid competitively a rehabilitation facility needs to be able to conveniently revise its layout to fit new processes that may become opportunities for the facility. Modern construction methods are capable of providing flexibility with movable partitions, or better yet with omission of partitions, and also with continuous sources of power as described earlier in this chapter.

PLANT LAYOUT DESIGN DECISION

A final suggestion to the rehabilitation facility planner applies to plant layout considerations as well as to many other rehabilitation facility considerations discussed in this text. Activity in rehabilitation facility development is increasing among colleges and universities across the nation, and the students of rehabilitation facility educational programs offer a planning resource for nearby facility projects. Even in institutions which offer no specialization in rehabilitation facility development, the students of more traditional academic divisions often have interest in and are capable of making a worthwhile contribution to the development of the rehabilitation facility. In one example observed, the students of a senior design course in Industrial Engineering were assigned the task of planning for a rehabilitation facility expansion to double the number of handicapped personnel served. Students were responsible for plant layout, materials handling decisions, equipment purchase recommendations, and overall justifications for a federal expansion grant application.

The reader at this point may be overwhelmed by the volume of questions to be considered in the plant layout of a rehabilitation facility. While it is true that the permanence of layout decisions increases their importance, it is hoped that emphasis of this point will not freeze the rehabilitation facility planner into inaction. The decision maker is often confronted with an array of alternatives, all of which seem highly satisfactory, or worse, with an array of alternatives, all of which seem to have significant drawbacks. A good plant layout, whether for a rehabilitation facility or for a conventional factory, is always a compromise. Necessities for compromise are compounded when dealing with a board of directors, many of whom are acting out of a strong sense of dedication to community needs. But once the important factors have been considered, it is important to proceed with the design and to get construction underway.

REFERENCES

1. Carson, Gordon B., ed.: *Production Handbook.* New York: Ronald Press, 1958.
2. Nadler, G.: *Motion and Time Study.* New York: McGraw-Hill, 1955.
3. Public Law 91–596: Occupational Safety and Health Act of 1970.
4. Salmon, F. Cuthbert and C. F. Salmon: *Sheltered Workshops: An Architectural Guide.* Stillwater, Oklahoma: Oklahoma State University, 1966.

CHAPTER 3

CONSIDERATIONS FOR DEVELOPMENT OF CONTRACT PROCUREMENT

MICHAEL M. DOLNICK

☐ Why Industry Contracts

☐ Public Relations and Contracting

☐ Factors to Be Considered in Contract Acceptance

☐ Acceptance of Underpriced Contracts

☐ Joint Contract Procurement

☐ Contractor Attitudes

ONE OF THE MOST PERSISTENT problems facing sheltered workshops engaged in contract work is that of obtaining sufficient work to keep their handicapped workers employed. Achievement of the workshop's objectives is dependent on an adequate work flow, and an inability to provide continuous and meaningful employment defeats the very purpose of the workshop's existence. Lack of work results in frequent layoffs and an accompanying loss in rehabilitation gains. Without a continuous source of work, client and staff morale deteriorate. When work is "stretched out" it is not possible to create the real pressures which are important in the development of good work habits and attitudes, a primary focus in the rehabilitation workshop.

This chapter is directed to workshop personnel responsible for obtaining contract work. Contracting is defined as the performance of work in a sheltered workshop to the specifications of the customer or contractor. The terms, contract and subcontract, are considered to be identical in meaning, and with some exceptions, refers to work not done on the contractor's premises. The important subject of manufacturing operations within a workshop is beyond the scope of this short chapter. For a more complete discussion of contracting, the reader is referred to "Contract Procurement Practices of Sheltered Workshops" by the author and available from the Superintendent of Documents, U.S. Government Printing Office, Stock Number 1761–0030. Selected material from this publication, to a large extent, represents the contents of this chapter.

WHY INDUSTRY CONTRACTS

Industry in general and companies engaged in the long-established practice of contracting require no proof of its advantages, having found it both convenient and profitable. However, an understanding of the reasons why industry engages in contracting is helpful in developing a sales presentation to be used in convincing a prospective customer that he needs the workshop's services.

Some of the principal reasons why industry contracts are:

1. Additional facilities and labor are needed to meet production requirements either on a short-or a long-term basis as a consequence of:
   a. insufficient work space or storage space
   b. inadequate labor supply
   c. insufficient machinery or specialized equipment
   d. emergency delivery schedules.
2. The work is outside the normal range of activities performed by the contractor and he hesitates to undertake a job that would interfere with his regular production schedule. These may be incidental or short-run jobs, or specialized jobs completely foreign to the basic operations of the contractor. In the latter case, it may be advantageous for him to seek a specialist with specific experience in the work to be done.
3. The contractor does not wish to use his skilled or highly paid personnel on jobs requiring a lower skill level and normally performed

at a lower labor rate. Also it is often found that highly skilled people do not like to perform unskilled tasks. Engineering talent may not be available or the contractor may not wish to assign engineering time to what he considers a nuisance operation.

4. The cost of contracting is less than the cost of performing the same operation on company premises. This conclusion is generally reached when a cost-conscious contractor is aware of the expense involved in hiring and training new personnel, in developing new items that include engineering and set-up time and the hidden overhead that always creeps in when new tasks are assumed, or in hiring temporary workers with a possible increase of the employer's Unemployment Compensation expense.

PUBLIC RELATIONS AND CONTRACTING

A year-round public relations campaign to keep the name of the workshop before the public is one element in a well-rounded contract procurement program. Such programs should include regular releases to newspapers, articles submitted to local periodicals, television and radio spot announcements, open houses and public speaking engagements. While it is not possible to correlate directly the effect of publicity on contract procurement, it is clear that it makes the work of the salesman easier. It is a mistake to expect a deluge of telephone calls offering contract work after the newspapers print a favorable story. Continuous newspaper, radio and TV publicity are merely necessary adjuncts to a program of contract procurement.

Most successful workshop directors recognize the need for continuous public education and publicity to increase the business community's knowledge of the existence of the workshop and the services offered. However, they also understand that publicity is only one aspect of the procurement process. Personal selling by workshop representatives is regarded as the most important element in an adequate contract procurement program.

One of the better forms of publicity used on the radio are tape recorded testimonials from satisfied customers. A TV interview with a contractor would be even better.

Direct Mail

Direct mail can be an important aid to a procurement program. However, it should be considered only as part of a complete procurement campaign.

There are many instances of disappointments where large sums were spent on a direct mail campaign and the results were poor. Direct mail is best undertaken during a workshop's formative period when it is soliciting contracts. Successful workshops have found that as their volume increases and repeat business comes in, they rely less and less on direct mail solicitation.

The following precautions should be observed in a direct mail campaign. If you are not skilled in the preparation of letters of solicitation, attempt to obtain the services of a professional. It is not unusual for a board member to think that he is a professional letter writer and some very bad letters have been sent out when workshop directors felt reluctant to tell their board members that the letters they wrote were not suitable.

The letters should be businesslike in nature, and appeals to sympathy should be avoided. Letters of solicitation may contain the following elements:

1. The services offered should be specifically listed; for example, packaging, electronic assembly, etc.
2. The benefits to the contractor should be cited.
3. There should be a mention of quality, production schedules and competitive prices.
4. A listing of some of the satisfied customers for whom work has been done.
5. An opportunity to call and explain the services should be requested. A written post card to indicate interest is a good idea.
6. It may be advisable to include a brief statement on the workshop purposes, organization, and employees.
7. A brochure describing the workshop and the services, if one is available, can be inclosed with the letter.

Procurement Brochures

The term brochure refers to a leaflet, pamphlet, booklet or advertising piece as distinguished from a sales letter. It is generally used as a give-away piece at the time of interview or as an enclosure with a sales letter. It is extremely useful not only for contract solicitation but as a public education device to explain the workshops services and program.

The contents of brochures duplicate to some extent the contents of sales letters. Brochures should tell the entire story to the prospect and serve as a reference for future follow-up.

Brochures generally include the following items:

1. A specific listing of the jobs performed in the workshop. Terms such as assembly, stapling, gluing, packaging, swatching are used.
2. The advantages and reasons for giving out contracts.
   One excellent brochure contained a check list as follows:
   No temporary increase in plant work force
   A fixed cost per hundred units
   No training costs
   No equipment purchases
   Factory space freed
   No hidden overhead or employee compensation charged
   No diversion of engineering talent for short-run jobs
   Relief from production pressures
   Extremely low spoilage rate
   Excellent degree of quality and accuracy
3. A listing of the benefits to the community resulting from support of the workshop.
4. The names of firms that had used the workshop for contract jobs.
5. Special abilities of the workshops such as quality control, prompt delivery and good workmanship.

In a survey made among purchasing agents only about 12 percent considered advertising to be an important influence in the selection of a source of supply. Generally they were not interested in institutional advertising, goodwill advertising or any type of advertising that did not specifically give them information that was of direct assistance to them in buying. Advertising was kept only if there was sufficient descriptive information on the product to enable the buyer to file it for reference. Many brochures fall short because they have large amounts of copy requiring a great deal of reading in order to get all the essential facts; they fail to be specific about workshops services and do not get the readers attention quickly.

Brochures should always be written so that they are directed to the reader in terms that he will understand.

In the development of a brochure, it is advisable to get skilled help. Quite often this is available as a contribution through board members of supporting groups. It is also advisable to involve persons familiar with the workshop and problems of contract work in the planning of the publication. The salesman who will be most directly involved in the utilization of the brochure should have an opportunity to assist in its development. Avoid rehabilitation jargon and give consideration to attractive layout and appearance.

The Salesman

All of the workshop's public relations activities are no substitute for the personal solicitation effort. Even positive responses to a sales letter have to be followed up with a personal sales call in order to close the deal. Most executive directors of workshops find that they can never get completely away from contract procurement. Even when they have full-time contract salesmen they find that long-time customers may insist on dealing with the head man. The best contract procurement results are obtained through the efforts of aggressive, hard-working salesman.

Good procurement men have common characteristics:

1. They have a thorough knowledge of the industrial community; they use their knowledge to follow the most productive leads; they develop a wide acquaintance with responsible company officials; they exploit their membership in business groups and service clubs; they keep abreast of industrial trends through reading, convention attendance and business contacts.
2. They are hard working; they believe that you have to make calls to get results and are persistent in follow-up when they believe that the company is a prospect for current or future work. Office preparation, telephone calls, direct mail and publicity campaigns may all be necessary preparatory work, but they know that there is no substitute for personal contact and aggressive salesmanship.

In addition, it can be said that the good contract procurement man knows and understands all aspects of the workshop program. He is not merely a salesman; he is the representative of the workshop to the industrial community. His effectiveness increases with his knowledge and understanding of industrial practices, his ability to estimate and compute prices and his ability to help the contractor with specialized industrial problems. Many workshops, recognizing the importance of good contract procurement men, have delegated to them major contractor liaison responsibilities after jobs are sold.

Sales Leads

A good resource for developing a list of prospects are the various industrial directories and the most useful are those published locally by Chambers of Commerce. Many directories give names of executives, products manufactured, size of company, number of employees and other specialized financial and background data.

Another frequent resource is the recommendation of board members. Many first contracts are obtained after influential board members open doors and pave the way for a sales presentation. In some cases board members have assumed the leadership in heading up contract procurement committees, have introduced workshop staff to industrial leaders and have arranged for guided tours through industrial plants. Board members have also assumed responsibility for underwriting costs of brochures or loaning members of their own staff for various forms of assistance of a professional or technical nature.

There are some negative aspects to too much involvement of board members. Some waste motion occurs when salesmen have to follow up all leads provided by board members and it is usually not good politics to ignore a recommendation of a board member even when the lead is known to be futile. There is also the danger of offending the foreman or production manager if he is told by top management to award a contract against his will. Sometimes inappropriate or impossible jobs may be awarded to show that the production manager has cooperated with orders to assist the workshop. Board members' leads that are most productive are those where more than just names and addresses are given. The procurement man should know something about company operations and products, duties and responsibilities of various key personnel and the person who has final authority to make the decision about contract work. With this type of information, the salesman has a selling advantage and can speak in exact terms instead of generalities.

All good contract procurement men utilize their knowledge of the industrial community to develop their prospect list. Salesman with specialized industrial backgrounds usually maintain their contacts in the industry. Memberships in certain service clubs is a way of broadening knowledge about the industrial community and may lead to contracts; however, most procurement men hold that only a "soft sell" should be used to promote a shop at a service club function. Awareness of general business conditions through reading of labor market trend data in newspapers and trade journals is also important. Attendance at various conventions of industries such as toys, pharmaceuticals, etc. sometimes provide useful leads.

The most difficult form of contract solicitation is door-to-door solicitation without introduction, appointment or previous knowledge of the prospect. This type of selling usually called "cold canvas" is often the only way a new workshop can break into the industrial community. It is time consuming and not often productive but if it is the only way to break into a concern it is still advisable to come in prepared with as much background information about the organization as possible.

When no industrial directories are available, the yellow pages of the telephone book can serve as a resource for the development of a list. Workshops that have purchased listings in telephone books report only fair results but it may be that these shops depend entirely on the advertising without supplementary procurement devices. The most frequently used classifications for advertising are "Assembly and Fabricating Service" and "Packaging and Filling Service". The classification that best describes the workshops services is the one to use, and a telephone representative can advise if the workshop wants to use this form of advertising.

Persons Called on

There is divided opinion as to the best person to call when soliciting contracts. It can either be a top company executive or the person in charge of purchasing. It should be noted that even though the top executive may be the person who makes the decision to give out work, he may not always be the right person to see. Most authorities stress that in large companies the purchasing agent is a responsible executive fully aware of the company's production and material requirements and is capable of determining whether a new product is of concern to his company. He should not be bypassed, not because it will hurt his feelings but, because it may violate sound rules of procedure and company policies.

It is not normal for salesmen to approach a new company and ask to see the President. The customary sales approach is through the purchasing department. Approach through top executives is generally advisable when the company is small and purchasing decisions definitely are not in the hands of a subordinate. Also, if the company has no previous experience or policy on the letting of work out of the plant, the first decision to subcontract will be made by a leading executive. The salesman who is able to obtain background data on the prospect's organizational structure and subcontracting experience, will be in a better position to determine the right approach to take. He is always safe in asking for the purchasing agent, but in many cases the sale cannot be made without executive approval.

Sales Presentations

A discussion of the most frequently used selling points will sound quite familiar because to a large extent they duplicate the items in sales letters and brochures. The following summarizes the contents of sales presentations made by successful contract salesmen:

1. a description of the specific types of work performed in the workshop;
2. work is of top quality and will meet contractor specifications and the workshop will not undertake jobs beyond the skill level of its employees;
3. deliveries will be on schedule, service will be good and deadlines will be adhered to;

4. price will be competitive; there will be savings in cost if work is given out; you can count on a fixed cost per 100 units upon which to base a selling price;
5. the workshop solicits that type of job that does not fit into the contractors regular operations;
6. on peak load activity there is no need to hire extra labor and then lay them off—peak load and overload work is particularly sought after;
7. the workshop has special skills in terms of both staff and workers and is particularly adapted to doing the kind of work solicited;
8. highly skilled labor need not be used on jobs that can be performed by lesser skilled persons; on short runs or problem jobs regular skilled employees may object and show lowered efficiency and morale due to disruptions of established routines;
9. the workshop is a resource to industry and should be regarded as a vendor of labor services;
10. the workshop offers outstanding supervision that guarantees quality work;
11. the workshop can offer assistance in engineering, manufacturing and design problems;
12. the workshop can provide extra space for storage and manufacturing;
13 the workshop has served important industrial firms in the community and their names are mentioned;
14. the specialized equipment of the workshop is discussed; contractors need not invest in new machinery;
15. prices and production figures on certain jobs performed are given as examples.

A frequently used term by salesmen is "nuisance work." Because of what it implies to the contractor, this term is not advised. The type of work performed in workshops is necessary for the completion of a product and to call it nuisance work detracts from the actual service the workshop gives to a customer. It undermines the dignity of the work accomplished. A better term for jobs that are necessary for the completion of the final product and which the contractors prefer not to do is "incidental work." Thinking in terms of nuisance work leads to the acceptance of a low or nuisance price. Thinking in terms of incidental work necessary for the completion of finished products results in higher prices for important work performed.

A statement that the workshop employs handicapped persons should be made in a factual way, but an issue should not be made of this fact nor should it be used as a device to gain sympathy. Many experienced salesmen caution against the use of sympathy as a sales technique because they know that this is not the way to promote the image of the workshop as a business-like resource of the industrial community. In a survey conducted among industrial customers of workshops the majority stated emphatically that the only sales appeal they would consider would be a businesslike one. There was sharp criticism of workshops who stated that work was badly needed and would be accepted even at a loss. A brochure is often carried and presented either at the beginning or end of the interview. Some salesmen build their presentation around the brochure. Another frequently used sales device is to carry samples of work performed and glossy photographs and sets of slides complete with viewer.

Number of Calls

There is no standard answer to the question of how many calls should a salesman make or how frequently should he call upon a prospect. Those procurement men who belong to the persistent school and who state that you've got to make calls to get results frequently cite cases of contracts awarded after years of continued calling. Persistence was, of course, on a selected basis because the solicitor felt the prospect had potential. These men also point out the factor of luck and of being at the right place at the right time. Many companies are in need of service only at certain times of the year, and it is only through repeated calling that the workshop may be considered since the majority of firms don't bother with files of emergency resources. Other salesmen feel that it doesn't pay to continue making calls after one or two refusals since continued calling could antagonize the prospect. Repeated calls are often not justified in terms of time and cost when related to results. A large number of calls is not always indicative of intensity of sales effort. Sometimes proper selling can result in a few difficult calls and there are salesmen who believe that the really best jobs lie with the tough customers who need to be convinced that if you get the job you will give it your best efforts. It was interesting to note that in a survey of contractors several said that workshops as a group are not well known and more frequent calls were suggested.

FACTORS TO BE CONSIDERED IN CONTRACT ACCEPTANCE OR REJECTION

If, in their anxiety to obtain badly needed work, workshops accept contracts that they cannot perform or are unable to complete on schedule, they run the risk of jeopardizing future business. The resulting damage to a workshop's reputation, when word of poor performance reaches the industrial grapevine, will more than offset the temporary advantages of full workshop employment. In determining whether to accept a contract, assuming it could be a profitable one, workshops should take the following factors into consideration:

Skill level requirements of both clients and staff
Supervision required
Production capacity of the workshop
Material requirements—whether furnished by the workshop or the contractor
Storage and working space required
Transportation and shipping requirements
Machinery requirements
Quality control requirements
Duration of contract—whether long or short run

Unusual contractor requirements or workshop deficiencies on any of the above factors merit serious consideration before the decision is made to accept or reject the contract.

ACCEPTANCE OF UNDERPRICED CONTRACTS

A term frequently heard in workshop circles is undercutting. Generally it has a derogatory connotation and is used to denote the unethical practice of pricing considerably below the prevailing market, rendering competition on a fair basis impossible. The exact price level where undercutting occurs is a matter of debate and subjective judgment, and thus it has been facetiously said, with some justification, that undercutting may mean any price charged by a competitor that is lower than your own.

Pricing below cost, on infrequent occasions, is well accepted in industry. When business is slow, industrial firms have been known to take jobs at far less than their usual markup in order to keep machinery in use and key personnel occupied. However, it is understood by industry that this type of pricing cannot continue for any length of time without financial disaster.

Personnel in workshops where unprofitable contracts were not accepted pointed out the following:

1. A price below the competitive market subsidizes the low-grade contractor and gives him an unfair competitive advantage over another industrial firm. The injured competitor has a legitimate complaint when he says that charitable contributions are given to workshops to support a program that subsidizes his competitor. In addition to inviting criticism from industry, other workshops have reason to complain. Low pricing tends to drag other workshops down to the level of the lowest pricing policy.
2. A low quotation in an effort to get trial business with the hope of raising prices later is very dangerous. Contractors resist price increases, and the consequent ill will caused by this procedure may offset temporary benefits.
3. Many contractors request quotations in order to determine the price of their own product. If the contractor's selling price is based on a low quotation, the workshop has an obligation to maintain its price.
4. A reputation for low pricing attracts only the undesirable contractors. Eventually all customers will be of the bargain-hunting type and higher grade industrial firms become wary of the workshop.
5. Acceptance of unprofitable contracts should be avoided. Extreme emergency situations may occur where acceptance of small short-run contracts at a low price may be expedient. However, every precaution should be taken to be sure that this is the exception rather than the customary practice.
   Occasionally jobs may be underpriced through error with resulting losses to the workshop. Such mistakes are not in the same category as contracts known to be underpriced and accepted because of a workshop director's desire to keep his workers employed. The newer and less experienced workshop director who may be over-anxious in this respect and prone to accept unprofitable contracts

in critical situations could profit by the advice of those who have had sad experiences. The possibility of continuing damage to the workshop's reputation and the danger of loss of support from responsible community leaders more than offset the possible benefits from the occasional acceptance of contracts that are known to be unprofitable.

JOINT CONTRACT PROCUREMENT

Workshops that are unable to afford full-time contract salesmen may find the pooling of sales efforts advantageous. In addition to the appeal of shared financial costs, busy directors of some smaller workshops are in favor of joint contract solicitation because it means additional time for them to devote to administrative and other problems.

Where a centralized system of contract procurement is in effect, it can be highly beneficial from the community point of view. The decision to undertake a joint procurement effort should be made in the light of local conditions and the individual needs of the participants. It should be recognized that multiple problems have to be overcome before the program will have any chance of success.

Where there are several workshops in a community interested in forming a contract association, consideration should be given to the following:

1. A clearly defined organizational structure, preferably with written by-laws and procedures. A board composed of interested volunteers as well as workshop representatives should govern the association.
2. A competent hard-working salesman employed by the association and reporting to the board. He should be an employee of the association not of the individual workshops.
3. A written statement of the salesman's duties and responsibilities.
4. Written operating procedures embodying agreement reached among the agencies covering:
   a. amounts of money contributed by each agency for support of the association
   b. methods of distributing contracts, and
   c. uniform pricing policies
5. Regular meetings of agency representatives to discuss progress and specific problems.

CONTRACTOR ATTITUDES

Many workshop directors believe that contract volume can be increased if employers would see the type of work being performed in the shop. There is the possibility, however, that a potential contractor would react adversely to the workshop if it did not coincide with his impressions of what a factory or production shop should look like. A contractor who is concerned with quality of work and delivery schedules may find the employment of handicapped people of interest, but he will not be sold if he feels the handicapped workers are not performing according to the standards he recognizes. If the shop does not look right, has been engineered by untrained people, and uses inefficient methods, it is quite likely that the employer will not be willing to award contracts because of a fear of poor workmanship and inability to meet delivery schedules.

Where the workshop has the reassurance of industry-wise purchasers of service that the shop will pass inspection, a blanket invitation to the industrial community may result in lasting benefits in terms of contractor education and new business. However, the workshop had better be sure that its image of itself coincides with the impression it thinks it will leave with the representative from the competitive industrial world.

Based on interviews with industrial purchasers of workshop services, it is evident that their primary interest is in how the workshop can fill a business need. They want sales presentations to be businesslike and straight forward, stressing the services that the workshop can perform for them. Appeals to sympathy are definitely to be avoided. As a rule, all contractors will give tacit approval to the purposes of the workshop but they do not want rehabilitation services to affect their delivery schedules or quality of work.

It is a common mistake for persons trained in rehabilitation professions to regard the techniques, terminology and operations of industry as of secondary importance to the purely rehabilitation function of workshops. The sheltered workshop is an unusual establishment that is both a rehabilitation facility and a business enterprise. It will not succeed if its management is content to overlook either aspect of this dual function. It is essential, therefore, that workshops adopt the techniques that their industrial counterparts have found to be productive. Workshops will have to accept the importance of aggressive salesmanship and reward salesman accordingly.

CHAPTER 4

CONSIDERATIONS IN DEVELOPING PSYCHOLOGICAL SERVICES IN REHABILITATION FACILITIES

RICHARD E. HARDY AND JOHN G. CULL

☐ Developing and Using Psychological and Related Services

☐ Indications for Psychological Evaluations

☐ Contraindications for Psychological Evaluations

☐ Referral for Psychological Services

☐ Selection of a Psychologist

☐ The Psychologists' Report

☐ Description of Models

☐ State Rehabilitation Administrators Views on Psychological Evaluation

☐ Results

DEVELOPING AND USING PSYCHOLOGICAL AND RELATED SERVICES

THIS CHAPTER WILL INCLUDE VARIOUS concepts concerning the development of psychological services in rehabilitation facility settings. The number of persons being rehabilitated at present through rehabilitation facility efforts has skyrocketed. Psychological services in rehabilitation must be

53

expanded and improved and this is a priority consideration in serving rehabilitation clients.

The rehabilitation counselor has been called the key to effective rehabilitation work and as such he is the center of activity, the coordinator and often the developer of services to his clients. The responsibility for the success of various steps in the rehabilitation process rests upon the counselor's shoulders —psychological and related services are no exception. The rehabilitation facility has become a prime resource for services for the rehabilitation counselor. No longer can state agency counselors do an adequate job in rehabilitating severly impaired clients without relying heavily on the services of a rehabilitation facility. Psychological services in the facility are no exception.

Psychologists are engaged in a wide variety of activities, many of which relate directly to the goals of the rehabilitation program. The rehabilitation facility administrator must develop professional psychological resources in much the same way that he develops community resources. Of the wide array of services offered by psychologists, three which the rehabilitation facility administrator will be particularly interested in include the following:

1. General psychological evaluations—relatively superficial but broad spectrum screening evaluation;
2. Speciality psychological evaluations—narrow in-depth evaluations (diagnosis of learning disabilities, determination of abilities, apitudes and interests, and description of personality patterns of handicapped clients;
3. Individual and group adjustment counseling.

Rehabilitation facility personnel are becoming increasingly aware of the need for making the most effective use of psychological services during the counseling process. Therefore, the new rehabilitation facility administrator should acquaint himself thoroughly with the services provided by the psychologist and the role each of these services plays in the rehabilitation process. He can then provide the most needed services to clients at the appropriate time in the professionally appropriate manner.

INDICATIONS FOR PSYCHOLOGICAL EVALUATIONS

Quite often the new rehabilitation counselor is in a quandary concerning when he should obtain additional psychological data. He feels, as a counselor, it is his responsibility to evaluate his client in order to counsel him. While he can agree on the necessity for psychological evaluation in the rehabilitation process, he needs some rather specific guidelines relative to securing such evaluation and the facility administrator can help in making this determination. The most obvious response to this question is, "The counselor should secure a psychological evaluation when he has a specific question regarding his client's personality or personal attributes." More specifically, the counselor should obtain a psychological evaluation when he is developing a rehabilitation plan which will be of long-term. If a long-term plan is developed, some basic assumptions are made relative to mental ability, interests, aptitudes and emotional stability. These assumptions should be checked out early in order to help insure the ultimate success of the plan. If the assumptions are not verified by means of psychological evaluation but are found erroneous, a great deal of the client's time and energies can be wasted. Similarly, if an expensive rehabilitation plan is being developed, a psychological evaluation should be obtained for almost the same reasons.

Many psychological evaluations are obtained at the beginning of the rehabilitation process during the diagnostic phase when the individual's eligibility is being established. A psychological evaluation should be made in cases in which eligibility is based upon mental retardation, functional retardation and behavioral disorders.

In developing the rehabilitation plan, the counselor needs to have a fairly complete understanding of the client's functional educational level, mental ability, aptitudes and interests. If this needed information is missing, it should be obtained. If part of the information the counselor has is unclear, ambigious or contradictory, the rehabilitation facility can help clear up the confusion with a psychological evaluation. For example, if the client has a reported educational achievement level or reported level of intellectual ability substantially lower than that required on a job the client performed successfully, the counselor should ask the rehabilitation facility to clarify the obvious contradictions by psychological testing.

If the counselor suspects important talents, capacities, abilities or disabilities which are unreported but have a bearing on the probable vocational objective, a psychological evaluation should be purchased from the facility to delineate these attributes. Also an evaluation should be obtained if the client has certain disabilities which later may materially affect his capacities, abilities, skills or personality. For example, a client who is experiencing mild anaesthesia in his hands and fingers should be tested for manual dexterity prior to settling on a vocational objective calling for a manipulative ability. A client interested in electronics assembly work should be tested for color blindness.

Lastly, a psychological evaluation should be obtained if the client is exhibiting or has exhibited behavior the counselor does not understand. If the client's current behavior patterns are not predictable and are difficult to understand, the counselor should enlist the aid of the facility psychologist to explain the client's personality structure. If the client's past history is filled with events or actions the counselor cannot reconcile, such as unexplained job changes, frequent moves from one community to another, a lack of organization to the client's vocational history and so forth, a psychological evaluation is in order to describe the client's personality structure in an effort to explain his behavior patterns.

CONTRAINDICATION FOR PSYCHOLOGICAL EVALUATION

Perhaps looking at cases when psychological evaluation is unnecessary would be meaningful. An obvious case where a psychological evaluation is unnecessary would be a client who has recently been successfully employed and intends to return to his particular vocation following the physical restoration and other rehabilitation services he will receive.

If the client has been successfully employed but is now unable to find similar work because of employer prejudice toward the handicapped, it is necessary for the counselor to use his counseling and vocational placement skills to convince the employers of the client's ability. In this case it would not be appropriate to obtain a psychological evaluation in an effort to change the client's vocational objective.

Psychological testing is not needed when a client has been successfully employed and the new vocational objective constitutes only a minor shift or the new job is directly related to his prior work. There is no need for testing when the client has developed a long and rich background of information regarding a particular industry or job family; his new vocational objective, though not previously performed by him, is sufficiently related for the counselor and client to be safe in assuming he can meet the demands of the job. A separate but related case concerns the client having a long and rich background of educational information and experience planning to study or work in areas related to his background. Evaluation is not needed in this case.

In essence, a psychological evaluation is needed when the client's behavior is to be predicted over a long period or his behavior is difficult to predict over a short period of time. An evaluation is not needed when the client's behavior is understandable and predictable or if he has established a related pattern of vocational growth over an extended period of time.

At times, counselors will threaten to deny rehabilitation services if a client refuses to submit to the testing and interviewing of a psychologist. In many instances, if the client continues to refuse, the case is closed—"This client is not motivated." Even though this occurs much less frequently than it has in the past, it is appropriate to discuss. As rehabilitation counselors become more professional and more aware of the needs of clients, they will be more attuned to the motivating factors operating in the client. If the client refuses services which the counselor offers, the counselor should seek to understand and modify behavior through counseling rather than being threatened and defensive himself and reacting in a punitive manner toward the client. The rehabilitation facility administrator and staff of the psychological services department can play an important role in this case by explaining psychological services to the counselor and assisting him in better understanding the client.

REFERRAL FOR PSYCHOLOGICAL SERVICES

When securing psychological services, the counselor should ask himself some basic questions and the facility staff should be prepared to answer them. These questions include: What specific knowledge can be obtained from the psychologist which will be of value in the rehabilitation counseling process? What data can he (the counselor) obtain and what data should he request from the psychologist? When these questions have been asked and answered, the counselor is better prepared to make an intelligent referral to the psychologist. As mentioned above, there are numerous types of psychological evaluations; therefore, it is inadequate for a counselor to merely refer a client to a facility for a "psychological evaluation." If he is expecting highly specific, definitive information from the psychologist, the rehabilitation counselor must set definite limits for the psychologist and provide him with the appropriate background information. Gandy's referral form if used will tend to increase materially the quality of psychological reports the counselor receives. This referral form should constitute the minimum information forwarded to the psychologist; however, generally little more than a request for an evaluation is sent.

Much of the information called for on the form is already in the case folder so it is easily accessible to the counselor. In order to select the appropriate instruments and interpret them, the psychologist needs the social-vocational-medical background information. Therefore, to facilitate the work of the psychologist and relieve the client of having to answer the same questions repeatedly and to increase the effectiveness of the psychological interview, the counselor should make a concerted effort to supply the psychologist all pertinent information.

REFERRAL FOR PSYCHOLOGICAL-VOCATIONAL EVALUATION

FROM: _____   DATE: _____
TO: _____

IDENTIFICATION:

Name of Client _____
Social Security No._____
Address _____
Sex_____Age_____Race_____Marital Status _____
No. Dependents_____

SOCIAL-VOCATIONAL-MEDICAL:

Economic Stratum _____
Family Environment _____
Formal Education_____
Usual Occupation _____
Vocational Success _____   _____
Leisure Activities _____
Physical or Mental Impairments _____
General Health _____

BEHAVIORAL OBSERVATIONS:

General Observations (appearance, mannerisms, communication, attitude, motivation):

_____
_____
_____

REASON FOR REFERRAL:

Statement of Problem _____
_____
Specific Questions_____
_____
_____
Enclosures: _____
_____

Note: This form was taken from Gandy, J.: The Psychological-Vocational Referral in Vocational Rehabilitation. Unpublished Master's Thesis, University of South Carolina, 1968.

An individual's economic status, home situation, the degree of vocational success he has experienced and the physical or mental impairments he has will have a direct and major bearing on his behavior and personality. Test responses and results have to be evaluated in comparison with the above factors. If this information is not provided to the psychologist, he will have to interview the client at some length. The more time he spends in this duplicative effort, the less time he has to evaluate the client.

The counselor generally has had several contacts with the client before the client is referred to the psychologist. Also, the counselor is a professional who is skilled in observations; therefore, it is of particular value to the psychologist to have access to the observations the counselor has made. These observations can be quite meaningful since the counselor sees the client under a variety of conditions and the psychologist sees the client only in the testing and interview situation on one occasion.

Perhaps the most important information the psychologist should receive is usually not given to him. This is a statement of the problem which prompted the counselor to refer the client to the psychologist. In order to specifically meet the needs of the counselor, the psychologist should have this statement since it will, in many cases, determine the particular instruments the psychologist will use. In conjunction with this statement of the problem, the counselor should outline the specific questions he wants answered by the psychologist. By considering these questions, the psychologist can further tailor his evaluation to the specific needs of the counselor.

Lastly, a good referral should include other reports, evaluations and examinations which have a direct bearing upon the psychological evaluation. These would include other psychological evaluations, social evaluations and reports, psychiatric data, the general medical examination report and some medical examinations by specialists.

SELECTION OF A PSYCHOLOGIST

After deciding upon what information the counselor himself will obtain and what information will be expected from the psychologist, the counselor has to select a psychologist. If the facility is to play an active role in the rehabilitation activities in the local area, the facility administrator must understand the basis upon which the rehabilitation counselor selects service components for purchase of services. The counselor can obtain psychological data himself or he may rely upon a psychometrist (an individual skilled in the administration and interpretation of psychological, vocational and educational tests; an individual trained at a lower level than that of a psychologist), a rehabilitation facility psychologist, a psychologist in private practice outside the agency, a staff psychologist or a consulting psychologist (these latter two will be discussed later). Generally, if he selects the psychometrist, the rehabilitation facility psychologist, the staff psychologist, or the consulting psychologist, the agency will describe the mechanics of referral in policy manual or procedure manual. The facility administrator should acquaint himself thoroughly with the policy manual or the procedure manual of the state vocational rehabilitation agency.

When the counselor is attempting to do part of the psychological study himself, it is very important for him to recognize his limitations in the field of evaluation. Certainly few counselors are skilled in psychological evaluation to the degree that they are able to use a wide variety of instruments. All counselors, however, should be able to use skillfully a small number of tests comprising a specific battery. When the counselor is inexperienced in the type of testing which he feels should be done, he must be able to secure the services of a qualified psychologist.

When obtaining the services of a psychologist in private practice, or in a rehabilitation facility, the counselor quite often will have at hand a list of psychologists who are well known for their competency and who are experienced in working with handicapped persons. It is generally felt that psychologists who belong to the division of clincial psychology, the division of counseling psychology or the division of psychological aspects of disability of the American Psychological Association will be interested in the field of rehabilitation and will be most helpful to the counselor. However, the counselor must recognize that psychologists, like other professionals, have areas of special interest. A psychologist who is knowledgeable concerning the emotionally disturbed or the mentally retarded may be relatively inexperienced in testing the physically handicapped.

When the client is sent to the psychologist, he is referred on an individual basis just as he is for a general or speciality medical examination. The payment is made according to a fee schedule developed by the agency and usually the state or local psychological associations or the rehabilitation facility administrators in the state. As with a new physician, a psychologist in private practice who is being utilized for the first time should be contacted. The counselor should discuss the vocational rehabilitation program, its goals, its procedures for referral, reporting, payment and the agency's fee schedule.

THE PSYCHOLOGIST'S REPORT

After the referral of the client, the counselor has every reason to expect and should demand speedy service for his client. This speedy service entails both a prompt appointment to see the client and a written report of the finding submitted. While the report should be received within ten days of the client's appointment, quite often it takes longer; however, if it routinely takes longer and at times exceeds three weeks the counselor should discuss the problem with the psychologist so that he may receive better service or change psychologists. When the counselor receives the psychological report, it should cover five basic areas:

1. Clinical observations of the psychologist
2. Tests administered
3. Results and interpretation of results
4. Specific recommendations
5. Summary

The observations of the psychologist are important since they provide the flavor of the evaluation and, without them the evaluation would be quite sterile. These observations will comment on the client's emotional behavior, appearance, motivation, reaction to the testing and so forth.

The tests which were administered should be spelled out for two reasons; first, most fee schedules are based upon the number and type of tests administered; but, more importantly, the counselor needs to know upon what data the psychologist is basing assumptions and making recommendations. In the reporting and interpreting of results, the counselor should find the results of all the tests given with an explanation of their importance. This section is highly technical, however, it should be very logical since this is where the psychologist builds his case. If some of the test results are not noteworthy or are not used in the diagnosis and recommendations, this fact should be mentioned and explained in the interpretation section. Essentially this is where the psychologist logically bridges the gap between his clinical observations, the test results, the diagnosis and recommendations he will make. Above all the sections should be very sensible and understandable.

In the recommendations section, the psychologist should make a number of suggestions which are addressed to the specific referral problem and the questions the counselor asked on referral of the client. Recommendations should be stated clearly and concisely. If the counselor does not understand them he should never hesitate to call the psychologist for clarification. The summary is a short, clear summation of the evaluation stated in nontechnical terms.

USE OF PSYCHOLOGICAL EVALUATION

After receiving the report the counselor is confronted with how to use the evaluation. The use of the data will be easier if psychological evaluations are viewed as an integral part of counseling and closely related to all other rehabilitation services and not as an isolated event or service. The evaluation can be used in counseling sessions to aid the client in better understanding himself and in identifying his major problem areas. Additionally, the counselor can use the psychological evaluation as a couseling tool to aid the client in developing insights specifically related to his relative strengths and limitations and in helping him in making reasonable plans and decisions.

In interpreting the test results to the client, the counselor should develop short, clear, concise methods of describing to the client the purpose of the tests he took and the meaning of the results; but, by all means the counselor should communicate only on the level at which the client is fully "with" the counselor. A most effective means of interpreting test results is relating test data in meaningful terms to the client's behavior. A trap to avoid is becoming overly identified with the client's test scores. They should be presented in a manner that will allow him to question, reject, accept or modify the presentation and interpretation without having to reject the counselor. The counselor should not project his own subjective feelings into the results he is using.

Cautions in Using Psychological Test Scores

While psychological testing plays a vital role in the rehabilitation process, there are some cautions which need to be exercised in their use. It should be remembered that test scores are just that-only test scores. The indications are a product of the interpretation of the scores. Tests are only an *aid* to the counselor; they should never become the prime reason for a program of action in a client's rehabilitation. They are too fallible. They are too susceptible to human error to be relied upon completely. While scores are valuable in indicating vocational areas which merit consideration, the counselor should remember that tests are rather weak in industrial validation. But most importantly, it should be remembered that the individual can adjust to several occupations. Inherent in testing philosophy is the concept that an individual is "predestined" to only one occupation.

Developing Models of Psychological Services for State Rehabilitation Agencies

As the scope and commitment of vocational rehabilitation has expanded to include services to the culturally disadvantaged and those with behavioral disorders, so has the reliance on and need for psychologists in rehabiliation work. Psychologists who are trained at the doctoral level and who are aware of rehabilitation objectives and procedures are needed urgently.

The number of psychologists employed in vocational rehabilitation is limited, in order to obtain psychological services on a statewide basis, many vocational rehabilitation departments have generally taken one of three approaches in developing models of psychological services. The approaches might be labeled as (a) the consultation model, (b) the strict panel model and (c) the supervising psychologist model.

DESCRIPTION OF MODELS

The *consultation model* is relatively simple in structure. The department of rehabilitation must develop cooperative relationships with psychologists who are employed by institutions and rehabilitation facilities or who are in private practice. Usually rehabilitation area office supervisors contact these individuals and ask that they serve as consultants in psychology to the vocational rehabilitation program.

There are some problems with this approach. Many rehabilitation workers are not knowledgeable about the selection of qualified psychologists, and many psychologists are unaware of the objectives of rehabilitation. Unless there is considerable effort on the part of rehabilitation personnel and psychologists to develop understanding, the relationship between the rehabilitation department and consulting psychologists can be strained. This type of working relationship results in complaints from rehabilitation personnel that they are not getting the type of information they really need from psychologists. In addition, psychologists may not become fully involved and committed to the objectives of the rehabilitation programs. In addition, there is often confusion about fees and the selection of psychologists for various types of work such as psychotherapy and psychological evaluation of clients with catastrophic disabilities.

The *strict panel model* is the second approach which is used by some departments of rehabilitation. In this model, a part-time state consultant in psychology is usually hired. The state consultant in psychology and the rehabilitation department, in cooperation with the state psychological association, selects a panel of psychologists which represents various phases of professional psychology. The panel rules on the qualifications of psychologists who apply to perform various functions for the vocational rehabilitation department and specifies areas of competency of individual psychologists. The state psychological consultant for the vocational rehabilitation department usually chairs the panel. Panel members develop a list of psychologists and describe services psychologists are qualified to offer to the vocational rehabilitation department.

This approach can be criticized as duplicated effort if the state has a certification or licensing board. Such boards examine the credentials of psychologists and determine areas of competency. The state licensing or certification board also is concerned with violations of ethical standards. The strict panel model can be very useful in states where no state board of examiners has been appointed.

The *supervising psychologist model* is a third approach which is used by departments of vocational rehabilitation. This model requires the employment of a full-time psychologist who serves as state supervisor of psychological services. The supervising psychologist has statewide responsibility for developing effective working relationships with other psychologists employed on either a full-time or part-time basis. He recommends psychologists for work with the rehabilitation department. He may also act as chairman of a panel of psychologists which meets to consider special psychological problems in vocational rehabilitation. The panel can also help in developing cooperative relationships between the rehabilitation department and consulting psychologists.

The supervising psychologist helps rehabilitation staff members develop understanding of concepts that will be of value to them in their work in vocational rehabilitation. He should participate actively in in-service training activities for professional rehabilitation staff members. He visits area offices and facilities in order to work with consulting psychologists and rehabilitation personnel.

In addition, the supervising psychologist assures that the psychologists working for the rehabilitation department maintain standards of practice in accordance with the laws of the state and with standards established by the American Psychological Association. He may also plan training programs for them in order that they may develop improved understanding of the complexities of vocational rehabilitation work.

These models and general variations of them have been used by most state rehabilitation departments, although some departments have not yet developed psychological services on a statewide basis.

Of the three described models, the supervising psychologist approach seems most effective, mainly because it allows an individual who is a psychologist to devote a substantial portion of his time to psychological services within the department of rehabilitation. A supervising psychologist should hold a doctoral degree in psychology or a closely related field. He must be carefully selected. He has crucial responsibility for the effectiveness of psychological services in an important statewide social service program.

STATE REHABILITATION ADMINISTRATORS VIEWS ON PSYCHOLOGICAL EVALUATION

The rehabilitation process relies, of course, upon a thorough understanding of the rehabilitated client. Counselors develop this understanding by careful evaluation and study of medical, social, psychological and vocational components.

According to Hardy and Cull (1969) the widening range of vocational rehabilication services, along with the increasing complexity of disabilities with which rehabilitation has become involved heightens the need for more comprehensive evaluation services in the rehabilitation process. Even though a high level of evaluation is essential to providing adequate services to the rehabilitation client, obtaining pertinent and topical psychological information has been a continued source of frustration to the rehabilitation counselor. Not only does obtaining psychological information present a problem to counselors who have difficulty locating psychologists to evaluate their clients, but the psychological evaluation of clients presents a challenge to the rehabilitation administrators who must plan budgetarily for the provision of psychological evaluation.

Considerations In Obtaining Psychological Evaluations

The dilemma of handling psychological evaluations is a topic of frequent discussion by counselors and administrators. A basic question seems to be how the rehabilitation counselor can obtain an adequate psychological evaluation of his client without paying prohibitively large amounts in psychological fees for the increasing numbers of clients who need this type of evaluation.

Rehabilitation counselors and administrators generally acknowledge that from their experience, psychological examinations are extremely important in overall planning in the rehabilitation process. A study by Sindberg, Roberts and Pfeifer[4] has confirmed this acknowledgment by indicating that, in terms of the usage of recommendations of psychologists, reports are definitely useful in the rehabilitation process. More than half of the recommendations of psychologists were followed completely or were followed to a large extent by rehabilitation counselors involved with the cases in the rehabilitation process.

Administrators Sampled

We, (1970), sampled reactions of state rehabilitation agency directors relative to satisfaction with psychological services obtained from psychologists in private practice and the use of rehabilitation counselors in obtaining psychological information. All state vocational rehabilitation agencies were surveyed during the summer of 1969; of the ninety-one questionnaires sent out, fifty-five or approximately 60 percent were returned. Thirty-two of the fifty-five questionnaires which were returned indicated that state agency administrators do not believe that rehabilitation counselors should be prepared to administer a basic battery of psychological tests. Of the administrators responding to the questionnnaire, 49 percent (or twenty-seven) did believe that rehabilitation counselors should be trained to administer interest tests, 47 percent (or twenty-six) felt they should learn to give aptitude tests, and 44 percent (or twenty-four) believed that they could administer intelligence tests with training.

RESULTS

All fifty-five administrators who participated in this study stated that private psychologists are their primary source of psychological evaluations. Almost half of those persons returning questionnaires indicated that their state agency had hired psychologists on a full-time basis. Forty-three of the fifty-five agency administrators indicated that they were generally satisfied with the adequacy of reporting and professional services offered by outside psychologists. The most often expressed reasons for dissatisfaction by the twelve agency administrators who were not satisfied with outside consulting psychologists were (a) reporting was not sufficient for rehabilitation purposes and (b) there was an unacceptable time lag in getting material from the psychologists. Agency administrators concerned with programs serving blind individuals stated that psychologists in private practice often were not trained to evaluate blind persons. The observation apparently supports Allen's [1] statement that less than 3 percent of all psychologists work in the area of mental deficiency and only 2.5 percent are engaged in programs for the physically handicapped.

A majority of the administrators (58%) indicated that rehabilitation counselors should not attempt to administer a basic battery of tests because counselors lack an understanding of the principles of testing and evaluation. Additionally, thirty stated that in their opinion counselors lacked the time necessary to achieve effective testing and evaluation.

In states that recommend that the counselor have a counselor's test kit for his personal use in evaluation of clients, the following tests were often recommended:

1. *Tests of Intellectual Functioning*
   Peabody Picture Vocabulary Tests
   Wechsler Adult Intelligent Scale
2. *Tests of Academic Achievement*
   Wide Range Achievement Tests
3. *Tests of Vocational Interest*
   Kuder Performance Record-Vocational
4. *Tests of Motor Dexterity*
   Purdue Peg Board
5. *Tests of Vocational Aptitude*
   General Clerical Test
   Test of Mechanical Comprehension

In some states, the Otis Self-Administering Test of Mental Ability and the Revised Beta Examination are being used in lieu of the Wechsler Adult Intelligence Scale and the Wechsler

Intelligence Scale for Children. The following comment from a state director on the Eastern Seaboard indicates the general thinking of state administrators concerning the use of a counselor test kit, "We feel very strongly that counselors should be able to administer basic pencil-and-paper tests requiring level B ^{2} competency and preparation. We strongly urge that they not become involved with projective techniques and complex personality inventories."

Results of this survey seem to indicate that about 42 percent of the state agencies are moving toward having counselors use tests to make initial screening judgments of their clients relative to some of his basic needs and toward gaining an understanding of the client. Also, it appears that these screening procedures being utilized by rehabilitation counselors are helpful to them in making decisions which concern whether the client should have further evaluation by psychologists or should be involved in extended evaluation. Since fees for psychological services represent a substantial portion of the case service budget in the state agencies' overall budget, it seems practical to screen many of these clients through the use of a counselor's testing kit along with evaluating other data from the social and medical areas which may be available in order to make basic decisions regarding the rehabilitation process for individual clients. After such screening, the number of clients referred to psychologists for in-depth psychological testing and evaluation can be substantially reduced. This procedure would seem to allow for improved services to all clients since much of the money expended for psychological evaluation could be spent on other case services and comprehensive psychological testing could be completed only when, in the counselor's opinion, it would be necessary for the rehabilitation of the client. As a result of this study, it is the opinion of the authors that agency administrators have confidence in their counselors and generally believe that they can depend upon them to make the complex decisions which are required regarding the variety of types of psychological evaluation needed.

In summary, it was found that almost half of the state agency administrators felt counselors should be equipped to administer interest tests, aptitude tests and intelligence tests; however, a majority felt administration time requirements precluded counselors' routine administration of a basic battery of tests. While over half of the agencies have employed full-time psychologists, the major source of psychological evaluations in all cases was from psychologists in private practice. Although a large majority of state directors were satisfied with this arrangement, the main dissatisfactions concerned the relevancy of evaluations to vocational rehabilitation and the time lag in getting reports from psychologists.

Effective rehabilitation work requires comprehensive evaluation of clients. Psychologists offer invaluable information to the total vocational evaluation effort. The fullest and most effective use of their services by state rehabilitation departments is of high priority. We feel the rehabilitation facilities can provide invaluable assistance to state rehabilitation agencies if the facility develops a strong program of psychological services which will answer the questions and fulfill the requirements we have outlined in this chapter.

REFERENCES

Allan, W.S.: *Rehabilitation: A Community Challenge*, New York, John Wiley & Sons, 1968.

American Psychological Association: *Ethical Standards of Psychologists*. Washington, 1953.

Cull, J.G., and Hardy, R.F.: State agency administrator's views of psychological testing. *Rehabilitation Literature*, 1970.

Cull, J.G., and Wright, K.C.: Psychological testing in the rehabilitation setting, *Insight*, 1970.

DiMichael, G.: *Psychological Services in Vocational Rehabilitation*. Washington, D. C., U. S. Government Printing Office.

Hardy, R.E., and Cull, J.G.: Standards in evaluation, *Vocational Evaluation and Work Adjustment Bulletin, 2* (1) January, 1969.

Lerner, J.: The role of the psychologist in the disability evaluation of emotional and intellectual impairments under the Social Security Act. *American Psychologist, 18,* (5) 1963.

Sindberg, R.M., Roberts, A., and Pfeifer, E.J.: The usefulness of psychological evaluations to vocational rehabilitation counselors. *Rehabilitation on Literature, 29,* (10) October 1968.

University of Arkansas: *Psychological Evaluation in the Vocational Process,* Fayetteville Arkansas, In-service counselor training project for vocational rehabilitation counselors in Arkansas, 1957, Monograph 3.

CHAPTER 5

CONSIDERATIONS IN THE DEVELOP-MENT OF A PUBLIC RELATIONS PROGRAM

MRS. GEORGE P. LOOMIS

☐ Public Relations In the Planning Stages

☐ What Image Should Your Agency Have?

☐ Assessing the Image Your Agency Has

☐ Communicating Your Image—Public Relations Goal

☐ Public Relations and The Board

A PUBLIC RELATIONS PROGRAM is a series of related efforts designed to create a particular and clearly defined image of your workshop in the mind of the public.

People are the key ingredient in every public relations program; this is especially true for a rehabilitation agency, where even your product is people. Therefore, it is vital to recognize that from the moment an idea or need for a workshop is translated into "Let's do something about it," people become involved and public relations begins whether you are ready for it or not.

In this chapter an attempt will be made to elaborate on five areas in the development of a public relations program for a new workshop, including:

- Public relations in the planning stages of the workshop.
- Definition of what image an agency should have.

- Assessment of the image an agency has.
- Communicating the desired image.
- Public relations and the Board of Trustees.

PUBLIC RELATIONS IN THE PLANNING STAGES

If you are starting a new workshop you will require substantial support from a variety of groups in the community. Development of this support through careful selection of a planning committee is a first step in organization; it is also the first public relations effort, and a crucial one. It is both good sense and good public relations to give serious thought to who will be asked to help. The future of the workshop may well depend upon the influence of those who are recruited during the initial planning stages.

When people of stature and influence in the community give their time to plan a new facility, they begin to create an image of your workshop in the mind of the public. By recommending the workshop, they commit themselves to the success of the venture. As the members of the planning committee and the Board of Trustees approach additional people for guidance and support, they educate and inspire confidence in their proposal, a project based on demonstrated need. People with a stake in your success move your program forward and launch your public relations program.

WHAT IMAGE SHOULD YOUR AGENCY HAVE?

Building an effective public relations program requires that you first define clearly what image you want your agency to have—what image it needs in order to function most effectively. This image should be consistent with the goals set by the Board of Trustees.

Think About Your Audience

To define your image, first give some thought to the people in whose minds you hope to create that image. It is often said that a publicity person thinks about his story, while a public relations person thinks about his audience. Why is it important to think about your audience? For example, even though the punch line might be the same, would you use the same words to tell a funny story to both a professor and a six year old boy? Probably not—in each case you would use the most appropriate words to get your message across. Your audience makes a difference not only in what you say, but in how you say it. Your manner while giving routine financial information to an accountant would differ from your manner while providing information on social services to a handicapped person.

Consider your audiences. How do you want to appear to them? *Building the image is the goal of the public relations program.*

Publics in Your Agency

Within your workshop are three "publics"—clients, staff, and volunteers.[1]

Clients experience your agency every day. Their view of the workshop is tied to their initial impression and welcome, and to their present relationships with counselors and fellow clients. Does each client participate in setting his goals within the agency whether they relate to training and a job, or to extended work in the shop? Are his work problems and frustrations handled in a way which helps him to grow in confidence and self-discipline? The sum of his experiences creates his image of the agency. Satisfied clients can be a rehabilitation agency's biggest boosters, a most enthusiastic public.

Staff of a workshop is on the public relations front line continuously and will project to the public what it feels about the agency, both as a place to work and as a place to seek help. For example, which answer creates a more positive feeling?

"No, your case just doesn't fit into our program." or

"I really wish there were some way we could help you, have you tried. . ."

---

[1] Rebel L. Robertson, "Public Relations for the Non-Profit Organization" *Lesly's Public Relations Handbook.* Philip Lesly (ed.) (Prentice-Hall, Englewood Cliffs, 1971), p. 227.

Is the staff "treating cases" and "developing programs" or *helping people?*

Your staff meets every day with clients, employers, businessmen, people in the professions, and referring agencies. Each group requires a different approach and response, but the pivotal issue is how the staff feels about the agency, and what attitudes and objectives it reflects.

Volunteers are one of the workshop's most important audiences. They are giving you a priceless gift—their time and interest. The volunteer's image of the agency will include feelings about the dedication and competence of the salaried staff, about how the clients seem to feel about the rehabilitation services, and how the agency appreciates the volunteer help. Your responsibility is to provide skillful supervision of volunteer activities. A dedicated volunteer who is made to feel needed and useful will be an invaluable public relations asset; those whose time is wasted take home a negative view of your agency and become a liability. Close on the heels of the volunteer work should come your private expressions of appreciation and public recognition, such as a volunteer of the year award or certificate for hours of service.

Publics Your Agency Meets

A rehabilitation agency communicates with many audiences or publics outside the facility itself. They include customers of the contract shop, other service agencies, employers, prospective clients, members and other donors, foundations, government agencies, news media, influential groups of the community, and finally the important Board of Trustees. What image does your agency want to have with these publics?

Customers of the Contract Shop should have a picture of your organization as one which helps handicapped people, but which also runs a top-flight shop—clean, businesslike and efficient. The orders are scheduled properly, executed well and delivered on time. Billings are sent regularly and the work is competitively priced. It is "good business" to do business with your shop.

The staff of *supportive social services* and referring agencies in your community should view your director and staff as leaders in cooperative efforts to help people. They should think of you as flexible in approach, as innovators in devising ways to extend service—not as secretive, obstructionist or jealous of other agencies. Your staff follows up quickly on cases referred to the agency. If your employees are working and thinking in a public relations way, they will project to other agencies an image of a facility which is vital, cares for people, and which is doing a highly professional job.

Employers who hire the handicapped should see your agency as a reliable resource. Your job placement personnel know their clients' skills and capacities, and do their best to find appropriate job placements where the clients can succeed. They do not "sell" a client by overrating his abilities. If there are potential problems they try to anticipate them with the employer.

Prospective clients and their families look to you for help. You want them to feel that your staff is sensitive to the needs of handicapped people and their families. Even when the workshop cannot serve them directly, these prospective clients should come away from your door knowing that your staff cares about their problems. Any waiting lists should be open and available.

Members and Donors. A vital public! People who support your program financially have already formed a favorable view of your organization. Reinforce that positive image by giving them recognition and periodic news of your activities. Newsletters or meetings, including annual meetings, give you an opportunity to put your agency's best foot forward. When you receive contributions, acknowledge them promptly, and send a membership card entitling the donor to some special privilege—a free lecture, an invitation to a tour and coffee hour before the annual meeting, membership in a booster's club. Always account to your donors at the end of the year by means of the annual report. And do not fail to recognize their contribution a second time by asking for their support again the next year. Your donor should be proud of what his money is enabling your agency to do for handicapped people, and should feel a part of your workshop's success.

Foundations which have supported your organization will look with interest at your financial reports, and also at your program reports. Have you performed the services for which their money was given? Have you evaluated the effects of those services? Do you keep the foundation informed of your progress even though you have not approached them for funds recently?

The news media should view your agency as a cooperative, active community resource, and as a reliable source of news and human interest.

The influential groups in the community should be represented on your Board of Trustees and your corps of volunteers. The image of your agency held by power groups will depend upon who among them is actively involved in the workshop, as well as by the results which can be pointed to with pride.

The Board of Trustees is a crucial audience. The Board members' view will be an amalgam of all those mentioned above. More about the Board of Trustees and their public relations responsibilities will appear later in this chapter.

How about your image with the *general public?* The man on the street? Rarely will people in the community know very much about any one agency, sometimes not even its full name. Your goal is to make your workshop's name mean *something* to as many people as possible, and for that something to reflect *positively* and accurately your activities and objectives.

ASSESSING THE IMAGE YOUR AGENCY HAS

If you are joining an agency which is already established, how can you find out what image that workshop has in the community? Will you be faced with a negative feeling to overcome, a positive image, or with practically no image at all?

One way to find out how people in the community feel about the workshop is simply to ask. Question your waitress at lunch, the gas station attendant, a clergyman, a teacher, a physician.

Call the Chamber of Commerce and the local newspaper. Check in with any of the publics the workshop has and listen critically to the responses you receive, to discover if any clear picture emerges.

Next, phone the workshop and ask for some information. Notice how cheerfully the telephone is answered and how easy (or difficult) it is to find the answer to your question.

Visiting the workshop will provide many additional impressions to add to your composite picture. A friendly greeting from a receptionist, an attractive lobby featuring a colorful display of products made by the clients, helpful personnel, businesslike atmosphere in the workshop—all put a "face" on the workshop.

The foregoing are superficial impressions, yet they are precisely the ingredients which combine to create a public image. One caution to keep in mind is that a shiny new workshop does not necessarily house the most professional and creative rehabilitation; nor do elderly and inadequate quarters preclude a bang-up job being done. People and the job they are doing make the difference. It is fair to say, however, that if the exterior of your shop, which is on view to the whole community, is run-down and in need of paint the public may be excused for thinking that you perform as badly as you look.

COMMUNICATING YOUR IMAGE—PUBLIC RELATIONS GOAL

If public relations is to be more than ballyhoo, and it is, there are a few solid building blocks needed to strengthen the foundation:

   * The only sound basis for a public relations program is a *job well done*. Whatever your job is, do it effectively, earnestly, efficiently. *Do* guide people into vocations for which they are suited and in which they can be successful. *Do* produce high quality goods in your workrooms, and deliver the work on schedule. *Do* maintain a clean facility with a cheerful, businesslike atmosphere.

* Then *tell* people what you are doing. While it has been said that virtue is its own reward, no prizes are won by the agency which does not communicate with its various publics, often, with truth and enthusiasm.

* People work for people—not programs. Your public relations efforts will be successful in direct proportion to your involvement of people in those efforts. A state governor, for example, recently spent several afternoons in a state facility for the retarded. He worked with the children, feeding and exercising them. His *personal* involvement, and the picture stories it generated, brought his concern for retarded people to the attention of the public far more effectively than any speech he could have made.

Be Visible

Communicating, the essence of public relations, can be done in a variety of ways, only one of which is "publicity."

Increasing the visibility of an agency is a proven way to strengthen the public relations program. A *slogan or a symbol,* used repeatedly in your mailings, brochures, and on billings and through the media, is a useful way to increase your visibility and bring your agency's name and purpose to public attention. "The Open Door Workshop—Helping People to Help Themselves" or "Ability Workshop—Where the Handicapped Serve You!" The slogan should be short and still tell accurately what your workshop does. Then repeat the slogan over and over. By the time you are tired of it, people will just be starting to associate it with you.

Tours will also place you in the public view. Church groups, social clubs and schools are often pleased to be invited to visit an agency for a tour. This provides their members with an enriching experience, and gives you an opportunity to show people in the community what your agency does. If your tour guide is knowledgeable, articulate and enthusiastic, he will communicate your message. An experienced guide will tailor his remarks to the group. For example, a group of businessmen might be most interested in how the contract shop pays its employees and how it works out manufacturing problems; student nurses will want to know about the therapy program and physical capacities testing. It is courteous to let your reception-ist and workshop supervisor know when guests are expected so they will be prepared to welcome them.

When you are invited to address a group at their regular meeting place, you can take a tour of the workshop with you in the form of a *color slide presentation.* Slides are inexpensive to produce, but worth their weight in gold. They can be taken by an amateur photographer (volunteer perhaps) with a 35 millimeter camera. With slides, your audience can visit your building and see your clients working both in your workshop and on the job in various industries. Your voice makes the show personal and adds enthusiasm, plus a theme and a message. Your presentation can vary both in length and content de-pending upon the group and their time limitations. After the slide show, invite the group to tour the agency itself!

Often the slide show can be used at the workshop as an introduction before a tour, recognizing that sometimes the guide may not want to make comments on the workshop floor or that machine noise makes it difficult to be heard.

An offer of a *meeting room,* with or without a tour, is often welcomed by local service or church groups. If you have ap-propriate space for meetings you might consider this as both a community service and another way to bring people to your door. If your building is barrier free, and you will hope that it is, it may be one of the few places where groups of hand-icapped people can meet for social occasions.

Your Annual Meeting is a perfect opportunity for your or-ganization to invite news media, political leaders, business-men, professional persons, your members and staff to see and hear what you have been doing. It is your time to shine—and deliver your message!

It is also a good time to translate your program into peo-ple—by *recognizing* your volunteers, or by giving an *award.* Frequently awards are given to the company which gave your workshop the most business during the preceding year, or to the employer who hired a number of your clients, or to a client who has been outstandingly successful in his rehabilitation program. Inviting a *prominent person* to speak at the annual meeting will often draw a larger audience, and may be of particular interest to the news media.

Without exploiting *clients*, it is often highly effective to include them in your program. One annual meeting of a school for children with profound hearing loss featured a dance recital performed in perfect time to music the children could only feel, not hear. The recital was televised and shown over a wide area as part of the evening news. Not only was it a splendid performance and a great story, but it also created a positive image of that agency, far more effectively than the proverbial thousand words.

Your *Annual Report,* distributed at the annual meeting, may be a simple mimeographed sheet or a sophisticated booklet. Whatever its size and shape, let it tell your story the way you want it told! It should outline your goals and objectives, tell of your progress toward your goals, list your activities, explain the source of your support (fees, donations, etc.), and explain how the money was spent. It should list your trustees, members and volunteers.

A *brochure* describing your services is a useful and effective vehicle for communicating and for increasing your visibility. You will find that even a simple mimeographed folder will serve you well. It should feature your slogan and symbol, give your agency's name, address and telephone number, the director's name and those of the Board of Trustees. You will also want to include mention of your affiliation with any national association or with a United Fund, and any accreditation you might have received. Your brochure can be distributed during tours, or given to any audience addressed by your staff. It can be used at the annual meeting along with the financial statement, and can be sent to cooperating social agencies and sources of referral. It is also a helpful handout to prospective clients, to customers of the workshop and potential employers of the handicapped. Some large facilities with a variety of training programs and workshop capabilities will need separate brochures for job placement and the contract shop.

Design and publication of a brochure may often be accomplished with the volunteer help of a trustee, parent or friend. If you have an offer of help, your contribution is to supply promptly the information (copy) you want included, and any pictures or layout ideas you might have. Do plan to check the final paste-up personally to avoid having errors appear in thousands of copies. A printer or volunteer may not catch the error if the wrong name is printed under a picture. The printer will be glad to supply a proof before the final printing run is made, and it is worth the time delay to proofread it carefully. If you have no one to help you with design and printing, some printers are very cooperative and will give you pointers like these:

1. Check copy carefully before it is sent to the printer. Errors in the proofs which appear in the material you submitted will be corrected at your expense.
2. Odd sizes and colors of paper, and the quality of paper, will influence cost. Each picture will increase cost.
3. Use the least expensive method of reproduction that will suit your needs. In addition to mimeographing, which can be done in an office, you might consider using a small offset duplicator.
4. Always get several bids on a printing job. You may be amazed at the difference between them. Ask for samples of the printer's work, and ask him to specify what services will be included as some printing companies will help with art work, layout and paste-up.

A *newsletter* describing the activities of your workshop is another means of communicating with the public on a periodic basis. Once again, you may choose the form of a short letter, or a published piece with pictures. It is fair to say that a format which includes pictures will have greater appeal and will therefore be more widely read. In any case, tell your story clearly, directly and above all interestingly. Human interest stories are top flight material—a rehabilitated client, still handicapped, but pictured at his new job expresses thanks for the help he received at your workshop. Send the newsletter to your staff, to clients, to referring agencies, other social agencies, and of course to your volunteers, donors and trustees. In a newsletter you can also thank volunteers, announce awards, publish profiles of your staff members, and define new programs.

Breaking Into Print

Even in the earliest stages of developing the new facility, and surely as time goes on, you will need to explore another means of communication—*publicity* for specific events. There is no way in which publicity can stand alone as a "public relations program," nor should a public relations effort be judged by the number of lines about the agency which appear in the newspaper. The judicious use of newspapers, radio and television, however, can put the spark of life into any public relations program and carry your message to a vast audience.

Of all the media, newspapers may be your most useful. Why, in the age of television, is this true? Hundreds of thousands of newspapers are sold and read daily, and once printed, newspapers can be read any time of day or night, whereas radio and television are "momentary media." If a person misses your radio or television announcement, he usually will not have another opportunity to see or hear it. A favorable newspaper story can be reproduced and sent to your membership along with a letter or an annual report, and you will be reinforcing the impact of that single item in the newspaper.

Learning to use the the newspapers to the best advantage is not difficult, but a few guidelines may make the initial job easier.

1. Discover what newspapers there are, and decide which ones can be helpful to you. Often overlooked are church, labor organization, foreign language and neighborhood papers, and industrial employee publications. Sometimes an item announcing a staff promotion will not interest a large city newspaper, but will be welcomed by the suburban press where your employee lives.
2. Introduce yourself to the city editors, who are the people making the daily news assignments, and to the welfare editors if there are any. Make an appointment, meet the editor, leave a brochure and extend an invitation to visit your workshop. You will have paved the way for your next call, when you ask that one of your news items be used.

3. When you have a story you would like to see in print, decide whether it is, in fact, *news* or a *feature*. News is what the public should or must know: storm warnings, plant shutdowns, remarks of business and political leaders. These news items are time limited, and cannot be used a day or two after they are submitted. By contrast, a feature is something which will interest or amuse the public, and may be held for several days before it is used: a human interest story about how a client turned his hobby into a business with your help, or a picture story about a group of volunteers at your workshop.

4. Several days before you would like an item to appear, call the city editor or welfare reporter. Tell him you are sending him a press release, and briefly describe the story. If your item is one the paper wants to print, a reporter may be assigned to cover it. The reporter will call you if he wants more information than your press release contains.

   Suggesting a photographer is acceptable when there are good picture possibilities in your story. Except for head shots of guest speakers or staff members, city newspapers prefer to take their own pictures. Local papers will frequently use yours if they are black and white glossy prints.

5. There are many books available on preparing press releases, so a couple of general guidelines here will suffice. First, include the five W's (Who, What, When, Where, and Why) in your lead paragraph, adding more detail further along in the copy. Second, keep it short, concise and direct. Short sentences and short paragraphs. Newspapers prefer that you stick to the facts rather than try to "compose" in a particular style. Nouns and verbs are excellent—look suspiciously at adjectives and adverbs! [2] Third, no professional jargon. Last, no headline is necessary. Newspapers write their own and like the top third of a page to do just that.

   On top of the sheet, put your organization's name, (or use your letterhead), your name and title, the name of the newspaper and the person on that paper to whom it should be delivered. Then type "FOR IMMEDIATE RELEASE." Almost never do you request the release be held until a future specified date. Skip one third of the page and type the release, double-spaced with wide margins. Complete a paragraph near the bottom of a page, then type "more" on the bottom of the sheet if you wish to continue.

---

[2] Lowell W. Carter, and Art Edgerton, J. Beverly Fellows, Frank W. Mulcahy, Helen Nussear, Allen Speiser, *Public Relations Manual for Workshops*. (National Association of Sheltered Workshops and Homebound Programs. Undated. page 10).

Head the second sheet with your organization's name, page 2, and complete your release, starting at the top of the sheet. When you are finished, center the word "End" on the next line. Below that you might want to indicate what picture possibilities there are to accompany the story.

6. Now your item is in the lap of the gods. You hope it will be used, but you have no control over whether it appears on the front page or the last. If the reporter calls and asks questions, your job is to help him understand both the story and your agency's function. Educating the public, including and especially reporters, is part of the job.

Tuning in to Radio

Radio is a vastly under-used medium and you can use it to your advantage. It is ideal for public service announcements, participation in talk shows, and discussions of topics which concern your agency. Unlike newspapers, all radio stations are licensed by the federal government and must give a certain amount of air time to public service.

Every radio station aims its broadcasts toward a particular audience which is identified by age and other demographic criteria. Ask each station what its audience is, and how many people are reached. Then choose the station which best fits your needs. Probably AM stations will be most effective for your announcements, since their listeners want the latest news and views and are most apt to be actively listening.

If you have an event coming up which you want to promote, try asking a radio station to help with the campaign. Whether your event is a march for money or an attempt to fill a theatre for a benefit, you may be pleasantly surprised to discover what a following some of the radio hosts have, and how quickly they can drum up interest in your cause. One afternoon of a popular host's enthusiasm can be worth a thousand public service announcements!

Radio public service announcements require very careful wording, since radio time is strictly controlled. There are about nineteen words in a ten-second spot, fifty words in a twenty-second spot, and seventy-five words in a thirty-second announcement.[3] There will be time for only one thought. In the first words, get the attention of your audience (Voters . . . Parents . . . Employers . . .), then phrase your message clearly, and end with a call for action (Call . . . , Write . . . , Vote . . .). Remember that a telephone number will take seven words, so you may decide not to use it in a short spot announcement. Keep sending these announcements to your radio station, where they will probably be used in rotation with others as part of the licensing requirement. The station will let you know how often your announcements have been aired.

Having someone appear on talk or panel shows can give your agency great exposure. You will want to be sure the person who represents you will speak distinctly and express his thoughts well. A thorough briefing on the message you would like conveyed, and facts or figures pertinent to the topic should be given to him a day or two before the program is scheduled. Then, be sure you are there in the studio to meet him or to take his place in the event he is delayed.

When you prepare biographical material for a panel discussion moderator, double-space the copy and keep it brief and informative. The host will appreciate knowing about each guest's area of expertise. Spell the names phonetically if there is any question as to their proper pronunciation.[4]

Television is Action

Television adds a visual dimension. When you think about television coverage, think of interesting action rather than what the industry calls "talking heads."

Television stations also must devote time to public service announcements, and you should ask that they use yours. A colored slide can be used alone, but it will be more effective when combined with an audio message. Only horizontal pictures can be used and they will need to be covered with glass for television use. A ten-second spot uses one slide, a twenty-second spot is best with three slides.

[3] Ibid. page 7.
[4] Ibid. page 8.

VIDEO	AUDIO
Slide #1—Handicapped young adult sitting alone in living room, looking sadly out the window.	Sometimes people need a little help . . .
Slide #2—Same person entering your workshop, being greeted by counselor.	Our agency opens the door to a new life . . .
Slide #3—Same person smiling and being handed first paycheck in your workshop.	You can help give Marie a chance to earn her way . . .

Be sure you include the name of your agency, and time the audio portion accurately.

The editorial time offered by some television stations is an opportunity to place your director or Board chairman on television to deliver a carefully prepared message, often during prime time. Launching a building campaign, asking for contracts for the workshop, or thanking people for support during a recently completed campaign are some suggestions for use of this editorial time.

PUBLIC RELATIONS AND THE BOARD

The Board of Trustees is potentially the most powerful public relations resource an agency can have. How can you, as a director, guide your Board into a position to realize this potential?

An Educated Board

Start by doing a superior job of educating the Board. The function of the Board is policy-making; sound policies are built on a firm foundation of knowledge. Therefore, education of the Board member must begin early and be a continuous process. When a new member joins the Board he should be given a tour of the agency and an introduction to its goals and activities. He may also be given a *Board Manual* [5] which should include:

[5] Robertson, Rebel L., *op cit.,* page 228, 1971.

Names and addresses of all trustees
Names of key staff people and their responsibilities
Names and jobs of key volunteers
Agencies, persons and companies who support work of your agency
Budget information and other brief statistics
Historical information about the agency
Statement of goals
Some "official" replies to questions which are frequently asked.

The new member's interests and profession will probably suggest a committee of the Board on which he might serve; he should be asked at once to join and to participate with the committee. Get him involved as quickly as possible.

Joint committees of staff and Board present valuable educational possibilities. When a manufacturer joins the staff to help solve problems encountered in the contract shop, for example, he is on familiar ground. Solving production problems may be his most outstanding business talent. Not only does your workshop benefit from his ability, your staff has the opportunity to watch him grapple with their problems and come up with a creative solution. The Board member, on the other hand, will learn that often an obvious solution can't be used because of the sensitivities or limitations of the clients; he will begin to understand the difficulties encountered by the handicapped, and to respect those who work effectively with them. It is necessary, however, that Board members remember that their work with staff should be carried on only through the director, and that any suggestions regarding staff functions be made to the director.

Board meetings present a unique opportunity for educating both Board and staff. Every Board of Trustees develops its own characteristics and atmosphere; as your Board begins to function you might want to encourage open and informal meetings. If top staff members attend Board meetings, a number of advantages accrue. The staff will know not only the decisions of the Board, but the considerations which prompted them.

The trustees who hear the supervisors report periodically will recognize these key employees and come to respect their abilities and competence. During their reports staff members would do well to include case histories from time to time— their success stories—for these are often the examples Board members remember to use when asked about the workshop.

A *bulletin board* can be used to display newspaper clippings, articles published by staff, or announcements of coming events. The clippings should always include news (even society page items) about Board members and their families, and of other people important to the agency. The director or public relations person should briefly mention the items as part of the Board agenda so that everyone present will know why they are of interest to the workshop.

Board Notes, a mimeographed listing of recent events in the agency are a good way to keep trustees informed. You can mention the graduates of your training programs, list staff travels and speeches, any honors received, memberships in professional societies, etc. Distribute these notes at Board meetings, and send them with the minutes to absent Board members.

Follow the trustee meeting with a supervisors' meeting, to provide an opportunity to announce all Board decisions which affect the agency operations. You can distribute the Board Notes here as well. This kind of meeting schedule allows you to discuss general administrative problems far enough ahead of the next Board meeting to have staff reports prepared if needed.

Public Relations Thinking

Promoting "public relations thinking" on the part of the Board will pay big dividends now and into the future. Public relations thinking involves both staff and trustees being sensitive to the forces of social, economic, and political change, and giving thought to the public impact of their decisions.[6] For example, an agency opening a new workshop in an inner-city neighborhood planned a "grand opening" benefit. A volunteer

[6] Ibid. page 227.

committee made tentative arrangements, which included de-
touring traffic during the early evening event. Realizing that
the neighbors might resent this inconvenience during rush
hour for a party, no matter how worthy its purpose, the trustees asked that the benefit take place in the central workshop.
A bus tour of the new workshop would be part of the program.
Another "grand opening" was then planned to include the
neighboring residents, thereby encouraging their cooperation
instead of creating antagonism.

As the economic, social and political climate in the community changes, so must the programs and policies of your
agency. If jobs are becoming scarce in the electronics field, it
is time to take a long hard look at your electronics training
program. It is poor rehabilitation and poor public relations to
train people for jobs that aren't there. Your Board of Trustees
can be a valuable economic indicator, helping you to move
with the times. As you and the Board share your information
and plan together for the future, you will be developing a kind
of decision-making process which recognizes the importance
of the needs of people and socio-economic change.

Helping By Acting

In what other ways can a trustee help the public relations
effort of a workshop? He can *identify publicly* with the
agency—making speeches, or testifying at legislative hearings.
He can *promote the agency privately* among his friends and
business associates—helping to secure contracts for the shop
or encouraging the hiring of clients. He can help the agency
to decide *where to appeal* for help, and making the necessary
introductions. It often happens that only a Board member can
take the initial steps toward a potential contributor or a large
corporation. He can *thank* donors and friends privately, even
though they are thanked officially by the director. This tells
the donor that his contribution has been personally recognized
and appreciated by his friends. Trustees who are educated
about the workshop, are enthusiastic about it, and act in ways
to promote it give a tremendous boost to the public relations
program of an agency.

One subject trustees avoid in conversation with friends is any negative aspect of the agency.[7] Every workshop will have some problems, and these will be discussed in the Board meetings. It makes good sense to concentrate in public on the positive features of the agency.

There are public relations implications in all decisions made by a Board of Trustees, and these decisions move the agency into the public arena. Implementing the Board's policies, a director can infuse a public relations point of view into the relationships his staff has with the people they meet each day. It is as simple—and as complicated—as that.

Public relations planning from the beginning, clearly defined goals and a recognition of your publics will help you give your agency the image you want it to have. Doing the job well, and then telling about it will focus the public's attention, and your own, where you want it to be—on you and the way you serve people. The public relations message in rehabilitation is "people helping people to realize their potential." Rehabilitation is the greatest product in the world and *you* are selling it!

REFERENCES

Carter, Lowell W. and Edgerton, Art; Fellows, J. Beverly; Mulcahy, Frank W.; Nussear, Helen; Speiser, Allen: *Public Relations Manual for Workshops.* National Association of Sheltered Workshops and Homebound Programs. Undated.

Abraham Jacobs, and Weingold, Joseph T., Dubrow, Max: *The Sheltered Workshop,* A Community Rehabilitation Resource for the Mentally Retarded. New York State Association for Retarded Children, Inc., 2nd Edition, 1962.

Orzack, Louis H. and Halliday, Harry, Cassell John: *The Evolution of a Sheltered Workshop for the Retarded.* the Idea and the Process of Implementation, 1957-68, Parents and Friends of Mentally Retarded Children of Bridgeport, Inc. Monograph #4 in the Pursuit of Change Series, July 1969.

Rehabilitation Newsletter, Provincial Coordinator of Rehabilitation, Province of Saskatchewan, Canada, June, 1972.

[7] Lowell W. Carter, and Art Edgerton, J. Beverly Fellows, Frank W. Mulcahy, Helen Nussear, Allen Speiser, *op cit.,* page 28.

Robertson, Rebel L.: "Public Relations for the Non-Profit Organization" in
    Philip Lesly (ed.) *Lesly's Public Relations Handbook.* Prentice-Hall, En-
    glewood Cliffs 1971.
Sheltered Worshops-A Handbook, National Association of Sheltered Work-
    shops and Homebound Programs, 2nd Edition, 1966.

CHAPTER 6

CONCERNS IN LABOR RELATIONS

ISRAEL KATZ

☐ Overview

☐ Structured and Informal Lines of Authority Affecting Labor Relations

☐ General Labor Practices

☐ Statutory Compliance

☐ Workshop Standards

OVERVIEW

LABOR RELATIONS IN SHELTERED WORKSHOPS apply to three groups of workers whose roles differ, but who affect each other critically whether operations are normal or stressful. These three groups are the handicapped clients undergoing short-term rehabilitative training or indefinite care; the operating staff consisting of shop foremen or supervisors, clerical workers, maintenance personnel, truck drivers and the like; and the professional staff including the workshop director and other administrators, financial and legal officers, psychologist, physician and nurse, directors of the various programs, client evaluation people and such other support personnel having one to one relationships with the clients. In smaller workshops the financial and legal officers, the physician and some support personnel are often part-time people on retainer rather than salary and are seldom considered workshop employees. Boards of trustees of sheltered workshops constitute a fourth group of people who influence labor relations, but they are not in turn directly affected by related interactions.

93

In general, where boards of trustees are as supportive of rehabilitation as they are dedicated to financial solvency, labor relations are enhanced.

The purpose of good labor relations is to help achieve a constructive climate for high performance throughout the workshop so that rehabilitation and care of clients may be continually improved and the workshop fulfill its service commitments to the community as well as industrial or business customers who place work to be done with the workshop and hire rehabilitated clients when they become placeable.

United States Department of Labor laws, rules and regulations apply to each of the first three categories of participants, but special variances in labor legislation may be applicable to clients as arranged jointly by the professional staff of a specific workshop with its cognizant Regional Office of the U. S. Department of Labor; the Regional Office of Social and Rehabilitation Service of the U. S. Department of Health, Education and Welfare; and the State Division of Employment Security or equivalent agency. The prevalent assumption is that while members of the professional and operating staffs are physically and mentally normal and are thereby members of the general work force to which established labor laws, rules and practices apply, clients have physical, emotional or mental handicaps, singly or in combination, that usually make them less productive than persons in the normal work force. In consequence thereof, clients may be given special consideration by workshop management such as allowances of long-term absence from work without risk of losing their jobs for reasons of illness or temporary withdrawal because they lack transportation, permissiveness in unexcused absenteeism and tardiness, tolerance of very low productivity, and compensation at rates below the established minima to reflect this lower productivity while keeping them on the active roster and providing them with uninterrupted rehabilitative services. Once placed in private enterprise however, former clients are paid at prevailing industrial or business rates, considered members of the regular work force, and subject to the usual industrial pressures and discipline.

By all odds, the overriding consideration regarding the purposes, organization and operations of sheltered workshops is the rehabilitation or long-term care of handicapped persons so that they may achieve a noteworthy measure of self-sufficiency in their daily living activities, upgrade their earning capacities, enhance their social relationships, and avoid institutionalization. Since clients have serious handicaps, often including mental deficiencies, they should be "sheltered" from undue physical and emotional stress, as well as sharp business practices against which individuals with normal intellectual powers usually can protect themselves. Even when clients hold collegiate degrees, as some do, physical or emotional handicaps may temporarily diminish their intellectual acuities. Thus, wherever the intellectual ceiling has been lowered by physical or emotional handicaps, particular care must be taken to safeguard the interests of clients and prevent their exploitation not only against undue financial benefits to the sheltered workshop itself, or an industry providing it with work, or by having them perform uncompensated labors for individual members of the staff; but also to prevent their physical or mental abuse by other clients or staff, the prevalence of degrading policies and practices in the workshop, and unwarranted invasions of privacy in the guise of therapy or research conducted by individual members of the staff pursuing special studies or graduate credentials that either do not bear officially upon the operations of the sheltered workshop or are not intended to be of special rehabilitative benefit to clients. Specifically, clients should not be subjected to unfair advantage or used as guinea pigs to further someone's personal goals.

Despite combined public and private support, sheltered workshops are usually dependent in part upon income derived from their clients' production. Without such supplementary income, many sheltered workshops would close or fail to perform appropriately. Yet, this form of financial dependence at times detracts from the rehabilitative values of workshop activity to the point where clients do not benefit fully from rehabilitative programs and are often prematurely exposed to the pressures and stresses of unsheltered industrial environments. Of course, clients about to be placed in industry or business must be functional on the job to which they will be assigned. For that reason, clients ready for placement should be separated from routine workshop activities and given special training prior to placement so that their productivities and quality of output may be enhanced without affecting the performance of other clients who have not yet developed placeable skills or emotionality. Trial placement on a job with industry, prior to separation from the workshop, is frequently an excellent means for evaluating a client's final readiness to re-enter the work-a-day world if such an arrangement can be made with a prospective employer.

Severities of single or multiple handicaps usually place early limits on a client's skills, intellect and emotionality. For this reason, various kinds of work should continually be in progress within a sheltered workshop and the work to which a specific client is assigned must be compatible with that client's immediate or anticipated abilities to cope with such work. In most sheltered workshops, there are some clients who must be considered "terminal" in the sense that, due to their severe handicaps, the likelihood of their being employed outside the workshop is poor. They may remain in the workshop indefinitely. Usually, such clients respond positively only to very simple tasks, but show little or no promise for productive rehabilitation. Much of their time is spent looking off into space or sitting quietly at their work. The application of work standards, training in good work practices and instruction in materials flow aimed at improving their efficiencies are largely ineffective. To further good labor relations with clients and the staff, severely handicapped clients who are unresponsive to intensive individualized training should be exempt from established norms of production and related workshop procedures. At best, the number of extremely handicapped clients should be limited, as their presence absorbs much of the operating staff's attention. For less severely handicapped clients, the thoughtful application to them of accurate work norms and realistic production schedules, generally applicable to placeable clients, can serve to improve their workshop performance and interactions with other clients as well as the workshop staff.

STRUCTURED AND INFORMAL LINES OF AUTHORITY AFFECTING LABOR RELATIONS

It would be unusual to find a sheltered workshop, or any fairly complex organization for that matter, in which the actual flow of authority, responsibility and accountability corresponded precisely with its management chart. Organizational dynamics, personalities as well as the educations and experiences of workshop personnel, contribute to differences in their perceptions or interpretations of labor laws and personnel practices that constitute sound labor relations.

Consistency in decision making and labor relations practices, even under identical conditions in a given organization, is uncommon. On the other hand, inflexibility in labor relations that do not take into account effects of interpersonal and departmental interactions, group dynamics, personality differences and nuances of differing workshop situations, are as detrimental to good business practices as are inconsistencies in management decisions.

In sheltered workshops, where intellectual powers are apt to have broad spectral spreads even among the staffs, it is important to recognize that an individual's ability to adapt to inconsistencies, cope with politics and swing with the punches, correlates highly with intelligence. Good labor relations are promoted by staff members and administrators who can take difficulties and inconsistencies in stride and rise above petty politics and grapevine gossip.

It is the responsibility of all staff members to be cognizant of each others' roles and discretely inform the proper staff member about any problems relating to that individual's clients. Moreover, with high turnover in staff and clients, it is essential for all staff members to remain continually updated in changes affecting the total workshop operation as well as their own activities, so that they may communicate effectively with others in the conduct of their operations. It is the workshop director's responsibility to encourage innovation in the work of staff members and establish effective lines of communication, authority, and accountability throughout the workshop so that all involved can interrelate constructively and adhere to decisions consistent with workshop policies and accepted practice. But, staff members must also work cooperatively with workshop administration to innovate in the area of labor relations practices, consistent with workshop policy and the law, so as to help the entire workshop adapt to changes in operations and client rehabilitative programs that reflect socio-economic changes in the community at large.

Yet, apart from organizational dynamics, it is the workshop's director who creates the prevailing climate that permeates every component of the organization and who above all else sets the pattern for its labor relations. An open, honest, thoughtful and dedicated director will, with few exceptions, set examples for fair treatment of all involved. A workshop director who is a creature of moods, withholds information, plays politics, has special alliances with selected members of the staff, encourages grapevine gossip, makes inconsistent decisions and seldom keeps promises, usually operates on a basis of fear, opportunism and exploitation of staff as well as clients. These two styles of leadership have admirers in the business world and among some members of the executive boards of sheltered workshops. Invariably, however, labor relations in the second case are deplorable and, in consequence, critically detract from rehabilitative benefits to clients and the professional development of the staff. Probably, the most damaging failure in labor relations occurs when clients become pawns in workshop politics, as for example in tugging between production and rehabilitation personnel, and are shortchanged in the rehabilitative benefits or care for which the sheltered workshop exists.

Grievances

Complaints by clients may be lodged with their immediate supervisor either against each other, one or more members of the staff, representatives of industrial customers visiting to check on work in progress, potential employers, or about conditions in the workshop. Many complaints arc valid and require prompt attention because clients expect instant remedial action and may react in unexpected ways if a complaint is not acted upon immediately. From the clients' viewpoint, there is no necessity that grievances be rational or even related to workshop activities. The crux of the matter is that client complaints, real or imagined, significant or not, related or not to workshop events or personalities, should not become bases for contention amongst members of the workshop staff; some of whom may have personal axes to grind. Frequently, in the heat generated by client grievances among staff members, the clients' interests are overlooked while staff members argue about each others' prerogatives, responsibilities and procedures.

Client grievances, however trivial, should take precedence over other business at hand, and not be dismissed, ridiculed, or put off by insincere promises of remedial action, even if complaints are judged to be imaginary, or are initially presented by clients to a member of the staff having no direct relationship to aggrieved clients. Members of the staff against whom one or more clients may have complaints should react positively to those complaints and work with the clients' immediate supervisors to remedy or mitigate alleged offending situations, practices or conditions.

Client complaints should be rectified at the lowest pertinent administrative level, and reported at the next general staff meeting as appropriate, but only in a circumspect manner, so that all members of the staff may learn of clients' problems and those members of the staff, immediately involved in the matter reported, may benefit from the thoughts of their colleagues. It is essential, however, not to discuss strictly personal information about specific clients at any meeting except where participation is restricted to the principals involved, and when the discussion is in the best interests of a client or member of the staff.

Appeals by a client, in response to action taken by staff to which the client takes exception, should be presented either by the client, if capable of doing so, or by the client's immediate supervisor to the appropriate administrative officer in charge. Workshop directors should become involved in the resolution of client grievances only when all other attempts to rectify a grievance have failed at lower staff or administrative levels.

It is important to bear in mind that inability to resolve all client grievances at lower levels should not reflect unfavorably on lower echelon personnel, as it commonly does in the worlds of business and industry. Sheltered workshops are for handicapped people, who must be handled with more than usual permissiveness and understanding, so that resolution of grievances is often difficult. The typical pressures and penalties of business and industry imposed on employees for departing from established lines of communication and authority should not be applied to clients, or to their staff representatives acting in their behalf, even under duress. Bear in mind that emotionally distraught clients must be given every opportunity to air their gripes, however ludicrous the matter may seem or time consuming the effort, because unattended emotional upset of clients can lead to serious consequences. It is difficult, indeed, to reason with occasionally unreasonable or unreasoning people, but extra exertions to do so are often the essence of good labor relations in sheltered workshops.

No constraints, whatever, should be placed on clients in their verbal dissipation of emotional energies. They must be allowed to blow off steam. It is also important to maintain appropriate surveillance of upset clients immediately after resolution of their difficulties to assure that their emotional storms blow over without subsequent adverse incident. Such followup sometimes involves round the clock surveillance to which a member of the client's family, or a friendly but responsible client, can be assigned.

A dissatisfied staff member should register complaints with his or her immediate supervisor. After due consideration, either a mutually satisfactory resolution of the grievance is reached, or the problem is transferred by the supervisor through channels to the appropriate recipient of the complaint if it is an individual other than the supervisor. In the event that the complaint cannot be resolved, the case may be appealed through channels to the director. A sympathetic hearing should be held, however stressful the issue, and remedial action taken within the constraints of workshop policy, guidelines, available funding or salary schedule. Even where a salary adjustment is indicated but cannot be made, a frank discussion of the situation may temporarily satisfy an aggrieved staff member.

Professional Development

Because salaries of professional staff are generally modest, in some instances close to subsistence level, frequent turnover of staff and the need for staff replacements are common characteristics of workshops with which directors contend. Unfortunately, many mistakes are made that add to the difficulties of maintaining effective operations even when underpaid staff members remain. Dissatisfaction with salary on the part of an effective staff member should not be translated by administrators into rancor or punitive action, nor should underpaid staff members deliberately reduce their own performance. Dedication to rehabilitation in the face of adverse conditions is an essential professional quality for personnel in the sheltered workshop field.

Directors have the responsibilty, however, to provide each workshop employee with a satisfying job, living wage, and growth opportunities. Salary adds or detracts from job satisfaction, but when the salary cannot be raised for lack of funds or undue distortion of the preset salary schedule within the framework of available funding, directors should help their staff members advance in position when possible or assist them in relocating. A chronically dissatisfied staff member, however able, is not a positive influence in a sheltered workshop. In making promotions, the administration must apply prescribed procedures of affirmative action as a legal responsibility and should be familiar with the legal requirements of such action.

Deliberate interference with a new job opportunity for a dissatisfied staff member, by giving a poor reference or taking other negative action, is illegal and exposes the workshop as well as its director to risk of sanctions and liabilities. Without a specific written request by a staff member for a reference to a prospective new employer, a workshop director or other authoritative administrator should only inform the prospective employer whether or not the staff member would be rehired. With a written request for a reference by an employee, or written permission from an employee to forward a reference to a prospective employer, any criticism of the employee must be supportable with recorded evidence, and even if the criticism were valid, it must still be objective and free of guile.

GENERAL LABOR PRACTICES

Dissatisfied staff and administrative personnel readily transmit their feelings to the clients and in the process reduce the effectiveness of workshop operations. Dismissal of dissatisfied personnel rarely corrects the conditions, policies and practices that may be faulty and leads to continued dissatisfaction. Essential elements that make for job satisfaction and good labor relations are a clear understanding of what one's job is, what is expected of the job holder, and compensation for doing that job at the prevailing rate in local non-profit organizations for people with comparable educational backgrounds, experiences and responsibilities.

A formal but brief job description setting forth the duties, responsibilities, limitations in authority as well as the principal measures of accountability and performance, can go a long way in helping staff and administrative personnel understand their respective roles and recognize how they are expected to relate to others. These job descriptions should be available for all to read, and they should be reviewed annually to accommodate functional changes, fill in gaps and eliminate undesirable overlaps.

In hiring new people or promoting personnel from within,

it is necessary to bear in mind that individuals who seem well qualified to handle a given job may not prove to be the best candidates for that job unless immediate expansion of the job's responsibilities were contemplated. Each job should present challenges to its incumbent so as to stimulate personal growth. Every job holder, however, is responsible to make his job grow and then to keep growing personally into that continually evolving job. As a job grows, it is bound to bump into other peoples' preserves, so that seeds of conflict are sown and the workshop director is apt to reap an undesirable harvest of complaints. The director must anticipate conflict in a dynamic growth situation and focus the energies of workshop personnel towards a deeper exploration of their present responsibilities and broader horizons for their rehabilitative programs. Properly directed, workshop personnel will deepen and broaden their expertise and, in doing so, will acquire an enhanced appreciation for each others' efforts that will serve to close gaps in function rather than create arguments about overlaps.

Personnel appraisals of subordinates by workshop supervisors and administrators are for the most part anguishing annual experiences that seldom accomplish their intended objectives of telling personnel how they are doing, getting feedback from individuals as to ways of improving workshop operations, planning for each individual's professional development and jointly discussing common workshop problems from different perspectives. Most workshops are small enough to permit an ongoing dialogue between subordinates and their immediate supervisors that hinge upon clients with whom they interact. Errors in judgment as well as breakthroughs in activities should be recognized and discussed as they occur so that details are still fresh in the minds of those involved. Under such procedures, annual reviews, where given, do not focus mainly on the most recent mistake of a staff member and do not wipe out what the subordinate feels to be an overall record of noteworthy accomplishments.

Workshop personnel should be encouraged to maintain a log of their daily activities, unusual experiences, decisions, goals and accomplishments. This data should be discussed from time to time with their supervisors or at their annual reviews. At such times, positive aspects of an individual's performance may be intelligently accentuated by the supervisor and negative aspects considered with a view towards making improvements. Quantitative measures of performance that are a matter of record, such as the number of clients rehabilitated and placed, or the actual increase in production that passed inspection, are difficult to dispute and relatively immune to bias. They should be the backbone of any performance review. Labor relations are further enhanced when written acceptance with comments of a performance appraisal by the subject is sent, together with the appraisal form, to the workshop director for final review and compensation adjustment approval.

There is considerable controversy among labor relations experts as to the meaning of compensation and the role it plays in employee satisfaction. Some experts believe that a raise in pay produces only temporary salutary effects; that most people want a raise, but will be satisfied by other tokens of esteem and hence with less money. In actual practice, the significance attached to money by employees is determined by the amount of time employers devote to arriving at an individual's compensation. If the employer makes an issue of salary, and particularly so if some people are paid well even though they are considered mediocre performers by many people in the workshop, money rather than tokens of esteem is considered by employees to be the ultimate indicator of an employee's value to the workshop.

Apart from salary and other indicators of administrative approval, workshop personnel expect fringe benefits that may add up to between 10 and 20 percent of annual salary. The order of importance attached to different fringe benefits varies with individuals depending upon their financial independence, age, health and education. For people under forty, the order of priority seems to be: paid vacations, educational reimbursements, contributory health insurance, social security, free term insurance, a group purchasing plan, disaster insurance, a contributory pension plan, and disability insurance. Some or all of these benefits, while costly, are generally considered part of the salary package by workshop personnel and are an important ingredient in good labor relations.

Eventually, almost all personnel leave the workshop for other employment. A dignified exit interview with the workshop director is a constructive factor in the maintenance of good labor relations with those who remain. Invariably, some or all parts of exit interviews feed back to friends of the departed and ultimately to most remaining personnel, who recognize that some day they will have an exit interview, and hope that the suggestions they will make as they leave may improve the lot of those they leave behind. In some instances, what a departing employee has to say during an exit interview constitutes an important message to management from many remaining staff members. Feedback from a less than constructive exit interview can do untold damage to workshop relations and operations.

Entrance interviews and orientations of new personnel are equally as important. New employees, however humble their positions, perceive themselves as something much more than mere marginal additions to the staff or administration. They deserve individualized treatment, an accurate description of their jobs, an idea of problems to be encountered in their new roles, a description of the clients and staff with whom they will interact immediately, introductions to other personnel and tolerant follow-on guidance in handling paperwork with which they will need familiarization over the first few months.

Staff Guidelines

All members of the workshop staff should have a copy of an employees' guide, provided in loose leaf form to facilitate updating. It should be written in simple outline form and free of legalisms. Additions should be infrequent and discussed at staff meetings prior to integration in the guide. Remember, new edicts are diluted by their numbers, so the guide should be kept compact and deal with essentials. It is important to realize that a framework for operations can become a cage with each additional bar to innovation and self expression. Sheltered workshops are young enough to benefit from new concepts and activities. The purpose of an employees' guide is to help workshop personnel do a better job rather than constrain their activities for fear of mistakes. Of course, it is essential to protect clients, customers and the workshop generally from overzealous personnel, but well-conceived innovation and experimentation, openly discussed and encouraged by administrators at staff or casual meetings, will usually produce gratifying feedback and results.

Staff Meetings

General meetings should be brief, regularly scheduled after client workshop hours, and attended by all members of the staff and administration. The workshop director should preside. An assigned substitute or the highest administrative officer present could preside in the director's absence. The meeting agenda should be sent to all staff members at least one week beforehand; consistent with a preset format along lines as follows:

1. Introduction of new staff and visitors.
2. Reading of the minutes of the previous meeting.
3. Continuation of old business.
4. Feedback regarding workshop activities from individual staff members.
5. Special assignment reports from staff members.
6. Committee reports and occasional special presentations by visitors or staff.
7. Discussion of client grievances and reports of action taken.
8. Discussion of rehabilitative programs in progress, completed or planned.
9. Discussion of production programs in progress, completed or planned.
10. Financial status of the workshop.
11. Statistical report on client numbers, categories, placements, etc.
12. Discussion of special problems.
13. New business.
14. New individual or committee assignments.
15. Announcements by director.
16. Announcements by other members of staff or administrative officers.
17. Other matters to be brought to the staff's attention.
18. Adjournment.

General meetings conducted without hidden agendas and free of conflict, although heated arguments may develop, are most productive in problem solving. Participants should be encouraged to express themselves completely without fear of personal criticism and subsequent adverse comment or action. It is the director's responsibility to draw reticent staff members into discussions. The purpose of general staff meetings must be to exchange views and information for the enhancement of client rehabilitation and care, as well as the effective operation of the workshop and professional development of the staff.

Personal matters, or adverse comment relating to specific individuals, should not be aired in general meetings, but discussed privately in the presence of only the persons involved. Where private matters may need to be carried over into a subsequent general meeting, the workshop director should weigh the merits of doing so discreetly with all persons directly involved and introduce the subject objectively for open discussion, but assuring that the discussion serves primarily as an educational experience in constructive problem solving and pertinent information exchange.

Apart from general meetings, divisional, departmental, committee, or specific activity meetings should be held as required, but preferably at times that do not interfere with workshop operations. Such meetings may be either structured or informal, but involve only those individuals that relate to the business to be considered. A greater degree of personal interaction is usually possible at such smaller meetings and the appropriateness of personal criticisms among staff members increases as the number of individuals present decreases. At all times, however, arguments and criticism should be objective and within the framework of overall workshop objectives, goals, operations and interests. Subjective criticism of an individual staff member should be made only in the presence of that staff member and such other persons as may be directly involved in the matter. Personal criticisms should not carry over into larger meetings or become a subject for gossip amongst staff or clients.

Impromptu meetings of staff members, or between staff and

administrative officers, should be private and informal. Care must be taken by staff members to assure that their posts are covered responsibly by another staff member while attending such meetings if held during regular workshop hours. It is essential, however, that such meetings be justified when called during regular hours, and that information exchanged during such meetings be acted upon promptly. Meetings held during workshop hours tend to drag and they withdraw staff from their clients. After-hours meetings have a built-in incentive for brevity. Workshop administrators are well advised to make such meetings brief and infrequent.

STATUTORY COMPLIANCE

Federal laws and regulations, applicable to labor and working conditions generally, provide the basic guidelines for labor relations in sheltered workshops. They take precedence over state and local governmental ordinances except where state law exceeds federal provisions (as they do occasionally for minimum wage rates) or where specific exclusions exist as in the case of state-operated sheltered workshops; in which case that state's labor laws take precedence. Staff and administrators of sheltered workshops must maintain up-to-date cognizance of legislation regulating their operations; changing their practices as necessary to comply with changes in federal and state laws as well as obtaining specific written waivers from those provisions of a law affecting labor relations and working conditions that cannot be met after demonstrating diligent attempts to comply with that law to the satisfaction of the cognizant public agency and justifying the need for a specific waiver from the law to that agency. Upon securing a waiver from compliance with controlling ordinances, sheltered workshop personnel are especially obligated to comply with the relaxed legal provisions of the law lest the privilege of continuing operations be compromised.

Applicable federal laws are administered through Regional Offices of the U. S. Department of Labor and the U. S. Department of Health, Education and Welfare. With changes in federal organizations, divisions of departments responsible for sheltered workshop activities may change their designations, responsibilities, locations and personnel. In general, different federal divisions of the U. S. Department of Labor are responsible for employment standards, wages-hours, federal contract compliance, and occupational safety and health administration. The U. S. Department of Health, Education and Welfare, and divisions thereof, also administer social and rehabilitations services.

Local telephone directories give current organizational arrangements in a given area under the listing for the United States Government. Since there is apt to be some variation in federal and state office organizations and their responsibilities at local levels, it is well for workshop administrators to be familiar with personnel in their local offices, help them maintain an awareness of workshop plans and problems relating to compliance with federal and state laws, and enlist the help of local agency personnel to secure workshop certificates and such written waivers from compliance with specific regulations as justified. It is important that all cognizant regional or local federal and state divisions of government be aware of waivers from compliance with federal and state laws in matters relating to client compensation, working conditions, rehabilitation programs and services, vocational safety and health hazards, and environmental pollution as regulated by the cognizant regional office of the U. S. Environmental Protection Agency. Labor relations within sheltered workshops usually suffer when interactions with cognizant governmental agency personnel are less than satisfactory.

There is little uniformity among the several states in their cognizant agencies relating to labor relations or working environment, although virtually every function exists and state personnel generally work harmoniously at local levels with their federal counterparts. State organizations that relate to sheltered workshops in matters affecting labor relations are known variously by such names as the Division of Employment Security, Commission for the Blind, Commission for the Handicapped, Health and Welfare Commissions, Office of Human

Services, Labor and Industries Department, Labor Relations Commission, Office of Manpower Affairs, Mental Health Department, Public Health Department, Public Welfare Department, Rehabilitation Commission, and the like. All of these authoritative bodies are found in some states and often bewilder new workshop administrators because the responsibilities of such agencies are not always similar amongst the states, clearcut, or free from overlap. Sometimes such cognizant agencies operate at county levels. Moreover, with the turnover of personnel of federal, state, county and town organizations, it is sometimes difficult to find people in such agencies who can furnish non-confusing information as to which agency is controlling in a given situation. It therefore behooves workshop administrators and their attorneys to be informed about the roles of each federal, state, county, or town agency in their locale, as they apply to sheltered workshop operations generally and labor relations in particular. Yet, apart from maintaining appropriate contacts with these public agencies, it is well for every workshop administrator to become familiar with federal and state laws as follows:

THE WALSH-HEALEY PUBLIC CONTRACTS ACT OF 1936: relates to the employment of boys under age sixteen and girls under eighteen in any work performed under a U. S. Government Contract to manufacture goods for or supply materials to the U. S. Government valued in excess of $10,000. Workshop service as a subcontractor on a U. S. Government contract may make the workshop subject to the provisions of this act.

THE SUGAR ACT OF 1937: relates particularly to labor of children between ages fourteen to sixteen. It provides interesting background to current federal policy for protecting labor against exploitation.

THE FAIR LABOR STANDARDS ACT OF 1938: as periodically amended, establishes the minimum wage rate for regular time at work and minimum compensation for overtime or other deviations from the regular eight-hour day and forty-hour workweek.

CIVIL RIGHTS ACT OF 1964: as subsequently amended—relates to discrimination in employment and training for reasons of race, color, religion, or national origin. Reference: U. S. Commission on Civil Rights, Clearinghouse Publication, No. 17, 1971.

NATIONAL LABOR RELATIONS ACT AND THE LABOR-MAN-AGEMENT RELATIONS ACT: generally applicable to business and industry involvements with collective bargaining and arbitration procedures. While not usually applied to sheltered workshops, principles involved may be applicable to workshop labor disputes. Reference: "Grievance Procedures" Bulletin No. 1425–1, U. S. Department of Labor.

OSHA (OCCUPATIONAL SAFETY AND HEALTH ACT): relates to workplace standards, machinery and equipment standards, materials standards, employee safety standards, power source standards, work process standards and administrative regulations. These standards are directly applicable to sheltered workshops and few waivers are permitted. References: General Industry Guide 29 CFR 1910, OSHA 2072, U. S. Department of Labor, Oct. 1972. Federal Register, Part II, Vol. 37, Number 202, Dept. of Labor, Occupational Safety and Health Standards, Oct. 1972.

WORKSHOP STANDARDS

Established to protect workers against exploitation and assure them proper compensation for their efforts, workshop standards, above those prescribed by law, are usually set after negotiations between employee representatives and employers. The statistical average of production called the "norm," or quantitative measure of work done per unit time that passes inspection, demands a specific amount of compensation. Piece work placed by industry should be paid at the going industrial rate, but deficiencies in meeting the allowable minimum wage must be made up by the workshop. Production on overtime or other special basis, such as working on holidays, usually commands a higher rate of pay. Industrial engineers may at times be called in to perform "time and motion" studies as an aid in developing norms. They observe employees at work with a view to making recommendations that will increase their rates of production and hopefully maintain or improve quality of output without undue burden on the workers. As may be imagined, at times, workers resist this kind of help. Production norms are seldom applied to employees on salary, although if involved in actual production, they may benefit from recommended improvements in their operations. Overtime work by salaried employees is seldom paid, in which case it is voluntary and considered as "casual overtime."

Even though clients placed with industry are often subject to norms negotiated after collective bargaining for basic working conditions with employee representatives, the proper purpose for "norms" and "time and motion studies" in sheltered workshops is to help prepare clients for placement with industry. Frequently, this purpose is not clearly understood by workshop staff and administrators. In such instances, norms adopted from an industrial customer's shop may be applied to most or all clients working on a particular project provided by the customer, but with adverse effects. Results of time and motion studies performed with clients should be used primarily to improve client productivities and instruct workshop staff in better production techniques, so as to enhance the total rehabilitative effort and help prepare clients for placement. If the workshop's income increases too, so much the better; but norms or workshop techniques established to push clients and raise workshop income without much training benefit to the clients, are inconsistent with the spirit behind the sheltered workshop concept.

Where norms from industry are not available for consideration or adoption, they may be set by workshop supervisors after measuring the productivities of several staff members over several hours of work. Such "inhouse" established norms should be reviewed or corrected if clients cannot earn the minimum allowable wage or the salaries to which they have become accustomed. Yet, if one particular client outperforms several others at a given task and surpasses an established norm by a wide margin, that norm should be reviewed to confirm its validity, but the exceptional performer should still be paid in accordance with the set rate. At no time should an established norm be changed because a solitary individual out-performs a significant number of people. Moreover, it is well to bear in mind that continued application of unfair norms, or the manipulation of established norms and compensation for benefits that do not accrue directly to the clients, are practices usually considered illegal and possible grounds for difficulties with cognizant governmental agencies.

Conclusion

From the foregoing discussion, it should be obvious that labor relations practices, while centered about the clients, are applied mainly to staff and administration interactions. When labor relations at these levels are satisfactory, clients benefit as do all others in pulling together to make rehabilitation effective. There are other concerns in labor relations that merit consideration, but the essential concerns were covered here, and the remaining factors will become evident in the course of workshop development. Whatever the concern, constructive problem solving will serve to enhance labor relations.

The purpose of this chapter is to convey to the new workshop developer a comprehensive impression of prevailing sheltered workshop organization and activities that impact on labor relations and that are in turn influenced by those relations. In general, attitudinal changes brought about by enlightened labor relations make it possible to continue the development of new and better workshops that provide their clients and communities with important human rehabilitative services despite the difficulties and frustrations that working with seriously handicapped people entail. Good labor relations, almost as much as rehabilitative achievements, make the effort particularly rewarding.

REFERENCES

Growth of Labor Law in the United States. U. S. Department of Labor, U. S. Government Printing Office: 1967–0 259–580.
Equal Employment Opportunity Under Federal Law. U. S. Commission on Civil Rights. Clearinghouse Publication No. 17, 1971.

Delivering Rehabilitation Services. U. S. Department of Health, Education and Welfare, SRS-116, 1969, U. S. Government Printing Office.

Production Standards from Time Study Analysis. Local No. 2 U.A.W.— C.I.O. The Murray Corporation of America, Detroit, Michigan, 1942.

Work Measurement in Rehabilitation Workshops, Stroud, Ronald R.: Technical Monograph Nos. 1 and 2, Regional Rehabilitation Research Institute, University of Maryland, College Park, Md.

Records and Reports in Rehabilitation Workshops. Lamb, Auburn J.: Information Bulletin No. 5, Regional Rehabilitation Research Institute, University of Maryland, College Park, Maryland.

Standards for Rehabilitation Facilities and Sheltered Workshops. Vocational Rehabilitation Administration, U. S. Department of Health, Education and Welfare, U. S. Government Printing Office: 1967, 0–256–890.

Training Requirements of the Occupational Safety and Health Standards. U. S. Department of Labor, OSHA 2082, Occupational Safety and Health Administration, U. S. Government Printing Office: 1973, 0–512–381 (68).

CHAPTER 7

CONSIDERATIONS FOR PERSONNEL TRAINING IN REHABILITATION FACILITIES

HARVEY C. DE JAGER

☐ In-Service Training

☐ Traditional Education Concepts Challenged

☐ Stages in Personnel Training

PERSONNEL TRAINING IN REHABILITATION facilities may take several forms. It may include training in partnership with career centers, vocational schools, colleges and universities; or it may take the form of independent training programs directed toward entry-level skills or increasing career opportunities. It may be outreach training designed to upgrade personnel presently employed in other facilities, or it may be limited to in-house staff education. Whatever the directions of personnel training, facilities can be viewed as learning centers for many levels of training, and can operate their own programs as well as function as adjuncts to other training programs.

Because of its applicability to all facilities, the discussion in this chapter is limited to in-service training or in-house education. Its goal is to identify the roles and contributions that trainers can play in facilities and present some practical discussion relating to procedures for personnel training in facilities.

IN-SERVICE TRAINING

In-service training is concerned with those activities which are designed to improve the effectiveness of the individual in the *position he now holds*. The need for on-going in-house education has become accepted as a proper and necessary part of personnel work in most forward-looking corporations and professional trainers are an accepted part of these corporations' organizational charts. The need has been prompted by such matters as continuous and rapid changes in theory and technology, skill obsolescence, more complex and specialized bureaucratic systems, ineffectiveness of learned and traditional methods and approaches, more realistic and viable relationships with consumers, community and referring agencies, and so forth.

Even more important, in establishing the need for current and future in-service training at most levels and in most facilities, is the fact that: (1) many facility personnel lack or have had poor training for the position they hold; (2) in-service training relates most directly and immediately to the delivery of services to clients; and (3) it is able to address itself to problems that cannot be anticipated in generalized training.

Unfortunately, a standard litany of concerns which almost daily plagues hard working administrators and boards of directors frequently makes personnel training a secondary or, even worse, a luxury commitment in many facilities. An examination of the roles and subsequent contributions of a training professional, either full or part-time, should begin to dispel traditional thinking on this matter.

Training Roles

Several clearly defined roles [1] and their subsequent contributions to a facility as well as to the field of rehabilitation can be identified for professional training personnel. These include:

[1] Gordon L. Lippitt, *Leadership for Learning: Training and Development in the 70's,* American Society for Training and Development (Washington, D. C.: Project Associates, 1970), pp. 18–21.

LEARNING SPECIALIST: This role may be considered the "basic" or "traditional" activity of professional training personnel. The learning specialist is skilled in the ability to use learning theory and methods to meet training needs. He is the teacher, instructor, lecturer, and discussion leader. He is the manager of the teaching-learning process. He identifies areas where training is needed and coordinates the training. He does such things as pre-planning and motivation planning to insure that the learner will learn. He bases training on the felt needs of the learners.

If the training function is to make a significant difference within a facility it must be performed by those who have the expertise in making use of the rapidly growing knowledge about how people learn and change. Indeed, the lack of a good understanding of learning theories and their application to training has discouraged many facilities in their training efforts. Because of his expertise in this area and the lack of it in other facilities, the professional trainer is in a position to make a contribution not only to his own facility, but also to other facilities which for various reasons do not have their own professional trainer or other staff member who possesses the necessary expertise.

INFORMATION COORDINATOR: "In this function, the training person in an organization or community must serve as a seeker of information, clarifier of information, synthesizer of information, reality-tester of information, provider of information, and as a communications 'link' in the organization." [2]

As a seeker of information, the training professional must know his facility. He must be familiar with its current status and immediate goals as well as its long-range objectives in order to plan staff training accordingly. He must learn from those in leadership positions what objectives and results in a planned training program are desired. This and other information is necessary to assure proper outcomes of the training function.

As a clarifier and synthesizer of information, the training professional does not hoard the information he has gathered.

[2] *Ibid.*, page 19.

An important obligation of this role is the dissemination of the material. The results are that the facility becomes more responsive: goals are clarified, long-range planning becomes more articulate, department objectives become more succinct.

As a reality-tester and a provider of information, the training professional again becomes the catalyst to administrators and managers. He becomes the "objective eye" to guide and assess new directions, changed plans, and stated objectives to insure reality and feasibility. He becomes a source of information and a "sounding board" because of his expertise.

The function of communications link within a facility is obvious from the previous discussion. The importance of the communications function has been discussed elsewhere.[3] It is worth repeating, however, that the lack of communication or gaps in communication appear to form the greatest barriers to better and brighter days in rehabilitation. The training professional is in a pivotal position to keep the lines of communication open among administration, management, department and technical personnel. In addition, he is in a position to keep communication lines open to meaningful and purposeful communication; communication which will make a difference within a facility.

CONSULTANT: This role is considered by many today to be the most important one of a professional trainer. In it, he serves as a problem-solving consultant to the administration and management of a facility. In relation to his own facility in the role of consultant, the professional trainer may be termed "internal consultant"; in relation to other facilities and organizations he may be termed "external consultant."

The role of consultant is a natural extension of the roles of learning specialist and information coordinator. Its development in recent years probably results from the constant change amid unpredictable circumstances in the field of rehabilitation and consequently in the facility movement. Certainly this role offers challenge to training professionals to de-

[3] "Perspective: Harvey C. De Jager," *News and Views*, Vol. 4, No. 2 (September–October, 1973), page 2.

velop their skills as internal consultants on problem-solving, decision-making, and organizational change and development.

An outgrowth of effective training programs and internal consulting is the role of external consultant to other facilities and organizations. A similar external role as learning specialist develops. Unfortunately, many facilities and organizations do not have the resources, the time, or the personnel to perform their own internal consulting and training. As a result, those facilities which have successful training professionals can make a tremendous contribution to the field of rehabilitation by allowing their staff to share expertise, provided expenses and a modest fee are paid by the benefiting facility.

ADMINISTRATOR: This role is almost assumed if the previously stated roles are viable. A professional trainer can hardly function effectively as a learning specialist, an information coordinator, and a consultant if he lacks administrative ability. A professional trainer should know the principles and practices of administration and supervision. He should know basic management concepts such as management by objectives, organizational dynamics, group dynamics, organizational controls, and organizational data gathering and reporting procedures.

Effective administrative ability allows the professional trainer versatility within a facility and the opportunity to make a larger contribution. He may be assigned new projects, departments which are experiencing problems, or programs which need change. Such experiences enrich his external consultant and learning specialist roles while extending his contributions to the larger field of rehabilitation.

PUBLIC RELATIONS PERSON: This role, like that of administrator, is an outgrowth of other roles—that of the external consultant and learning specialist roles with other facilities and organizations. Because of his exposure, it is natural that the professional trainer is frequently viewed as integral to the overall public relations of a facility. This may be especially true with regard to the field of rehabilitation. While other staff members of the same facility are usually limited in their exposure by position and responsibility, frequently the professional trainer moves more freely and widely. Consequently, he, more than anyone else, is the representative and reflects the facility to the rehabilitation movement.

TRADITIONAL EDUCATION CONCEPTS CHALLENGED

Having identified the roles of the professional trainer and their subsequent contributions, we now address the more traditional and practical procedures of in-service personnel training within a facility.

Before a discussion of practical procedures is begun, it is important to challenge some traditional thinking in educational circles. De Jager has cautioned that three traditional concepts of education will need to be altered or ignored if significance, legitimacy, and credibility are to be given to personnel training within facilities.[4] Two of these concepts, the distinction between education and training and the distinction between professional and nonprofessional, are apropos to the present discussion.

First, the distinction between education and training must be discarded inasmuch as both are concerned with the process of human learning. The distinction has been that "training is narrow in scope and involves only learning that is directly related to job performance, while education is concerned with the total human being and his insights into, and understanding of, his entire world." [5]

We must move beyond this long-standing argument. The outcomes of educational activities must be of foremost importance as we look at staff training and development. How and where these outcomes can be best assured are the essential questions; the nonessentials are to argue training versus education in relation to the "how" and classroom versus facility in relation to the "where." We must concern ourselves with

---

[4] Harvey C. De Jager, "The Future of Rehabilitation Personnel Training in Facilities," in *The Role of Facilities in Training Rehabilitation Personnel*, ed. James E. Trela (Cleveland: Vocational Guidance and Rehabilitation Services, 1973), pp. 183–196.

[5] Leslie E. This and Gordon L. Lippitt, "Learning Theories and Training—An Overview of Learning Theory Implications for the Training Director," *Training and Development Journal*, Vol. 20, No. 4 (April–May, 1966).

the process of human learning—realizing that this process occurs in training as well as in education and in the facility as well as in the classroom. Unless this is believed, training will falter.

A second traditional concept of education which needs to be altered or ignored when contemplating personnel training within a facility is the distinction between professional and nonprofessional (or para-professional or sub-professional), skilled and nonskilled, trained and untrained, and so forth.

If training is to receive respect we must be prepared to accept a new type of rehabilitation personnel as professional; those whose credentials will consist of demonstrated competency in performing their jobs rather than the completion of traditional training and education patterns, either nondegree or degree.

Accepting the concepts that human learning occurs in training as well as in education, and that training is to be geared to meet facility personnel's needs no matter what their educational credentials may be, a discussion of practical procedures follows.

In the past it has generally been assumed that primary training of facility personnel should occur prior to employment. The presence of basic skills enabling the employee to perform a specific task have been expected. Although this assumption probably is still true, it is equally true that many people in rehabilitation are trained in other fields, or untrained, or trained inappropriately. A recent national conference has challenged the traditional training arena of rehabilitation personnel and especially recommended an expanding role for facilities in training.[6]

Assuming primary training is acquired prior to employment, supplementary training is still essential. Each facility has its own expectations from employees. Each has its own work environment with its peculiar procedures and methods. The rehabilitation delivery system model differs from facility to facility. Each facility has its own goals to which staff members

[6] James E. Trela (ed.), *The Role of Facilities in Training Rehabilitation Personnel* (Cleveland: Vocational Guidance and Rehabilitation Services, 1973).

must be attuned. Furthermore, training is a compliment to any staff because it means the administration and board of directors have faith in their ability to learn, change and grow. It demonstrates confidence in the staff's potential. It assumes a healthy restlessness and dissatisfaction. Indeed, training is the antithesis of complacency and the antidote to stagnation.

STAGES IN PERSONNEL TRAINING

There are really three stages in an in-service staff development and training program. An understanding of these should help administrators and boards of directors of new and developing facilities make meaningful decisions concerning such training in their facilities. Kozoll and Ulmer have identified and described these stages as:

Orientation: This is what everyone seems to do very well. The only difficulty is that a lot of information is usually squeezed into a short period of time or, on the negative side, extended over too long a period. (Sometimes even a week.) It's like trying to introduce the new member of staff to everyone the first morning on the job; the new staff member will inevitably forget most of the names and feel inadequate, as a result. When you think about orientation planning, your thoughts should go to those elements which are absolutely necessary for a new member of staff to know before he or she starts a job. When you list those ten or twelve difference points, assign a priority order to each and then pick the top three or perhaps four. These should be used as the elements in the first orientation. The others can then be stretched over the first two to three weeks, and related directly to the job they are doing. With one new item introduced at a time, there is much greater likelihood of a procedure, practice or regulation being absorbed and digested.

Initial Training: There is an obvious overlap between what goes on in the orientation phase and what is initial training. An arbitrary division can occur between those items which are given to a person before they actually begin working and other elements which can be introduced when the job starts. There are two essential elements in this phase of staff development: first, a slow step-by-step process of introducing only one new item, procedure or method at a time (and these are closely related to what is done on the job); and second, recognition closely tied to the introduction of any new procedure providing a base of confidence from which to depart when trying something new.

There is another element to consider which orientation should stimulate and this is the desire of new staff to ask legitimate questions when they have doubt in their minds. From the first day, you set the tone concerning questions by the way in which you encourage and accept them. Again remember, training does not have to be telescoped into that first period of time when a person starts a job. Problems may appear immediately but more often it is advisable to wait and let evolve.

Ongoing Training: This is where most everyone seems to stumble. It's easy to do a good job with orientation, because there is so much basic data to get across. The same holds true, though to a lesser extent, with the initial training—the staff member is new and will ask a good many questions. But after the person spends some time in the organization, it's easy to forget him/her. The unfortunate assumption is that if you don't hear noise or complaints, things are just fine and there is little need for follow-up training.

There is another reason why ongoing training tends to be the weakest area of in-service development. Relevant follow-up training demands that a supervisor or coordinator visit staff on the job and make some determination, with the staff preferably, of the types of growth-oriented training needed. Regular visitation and sharing of reactions among staff are all time consuming and are quite easily forgotten, once an administrator feels that a staff member can operate on his/her own.[7]

Practical Procedures in Personnel Training

The practical procedures covering orientation, initial and ongoing training are numerous and varied. A complete presentation is impractical and unnecessary. A limited discussion should stimulate thinking and provide insights into procedures in personnel training.

Orientation training begins in the pre-employment interview or perhaps in an earlier correspondence. Here is where the first building block in the possible employer/employee working relationship is laid. Needs, expectations, objectives and philosophies are expressed and compared. Compatability and commonality are examined.

Orientation training of a prospective or new employee should be carefully planned, should progress along priority

[7] Charles E. Kozoll and Curtis Ulmer, *In-Service Training: Philosopy, Processes, and Operational Techniques* (Englewood Cliffs, Prentice-Hall, 1972), pp. 19–21.

needs, and should be appropriately paced. All available literature concerning the facility should be given to an employee
before he comes on board. A history, a scrapbook of news
clippings, and the facility's publications, if available, are excellent orientation material.

Orientation training may include a tour of the facility, a slide
presentation, and an opportunity to visit with other staff and
in other departments. Much overall agency orientation will
have to be repeated after the employee "settles in." The primary concern of a new employee is himself and how he is
being assessed. Thus, major and initial orientation efforts
should center on those aspects of the facility relating most
directly to the employee. Orientation may and should be expanded throughout the facility when the employee demonstrates readiness.

Frequently overlooked in orientation training is familiarization of new staff with the philosophy, commitment and objectives of the specific department in which they work as well as
the total facility. Such oversight may result in employees really
never feeling a part of their department or the facility. Commitment to the handicapped and dedication to their job may
suffer. Again, this type of training, like others, must be appropriately paced.

Training relating to the specific job an employee does is
referred to as on-the-job training. Good on-the-job training
frequently makes the difference between an average or an
excellent employee. Most new employees need close supervision and guidance as they fit into their new roles and functions
and as their jobs are fitted to their individual persons. Allowing
this just to happen is to gamble with efficiency, productivity
and job satisfaction. Time spent with new employees will have
lasting payoffs if properly planned and executed.

When common tasks, needs and goals are involved, a group
approach to training is feasible. However, it is imperative that
commonality be assured. It is equally important that the
group's size be appropriate to the training purpose and approach. The lecture approach may be appropriate in present-
ing a new facility policy to all staff members; whereas a demonstration and practice session may be more appropriate when

training a limited number of personnel in report-writing skills.

Methods used in group training need to be selective. No one training method fills the bill all the time. There are many occasions when a combination of methods is called for. It is important to review the training methods options, considering the advantages and disadvantages of each type. Some common methods are: lecture, demonstration, conference, role playing, meeting, written instructions and oral directions. A growing mass of audio and visual material is becoming available to enrich and expand training methods.

All training, especially group training, should be developed from the content to be covered, then the best form in which to present that content, and finally the best people to do it.[8] Starting from the opposite end limits training immediately by the personnel who perform it. It is not necessary that all training be conducted by professional trainers. Many staff members can make an effective contribution within the framework of a total facility training program.

There are numerous techniques which expedite individual and group training. One is timing which relates to the need for the training as well as the scheduling of it. Prompt starting and termination times are basic. A dragged-out, dragged-on training session is the last thing most staff members care to tolerate. Keeping in mind that training is an ongoing process, it is essential that each event be well-planned, properly executed and amply brief. The first or last one-half hour of a day works well. Usually clients are not in the building, thus freeing most staff. These times of day also assure a brief session with a fixed termination time. Lunch hours may be used for more casual and informal training. Movies with strong appeal are especially effective during lunch periods because they allow a comfortable dining setting in a relaxed atmosphere as well as an opportunity to learn. Circulation of carefully selected news clippings, articles, manuals and books within a department or to selected personnel such as counselors or production supervisors is purposeful.

Out-service training, that is, training of staff outside of their

[8] *Ibid.,* page 46.

own facility, should not be overlooked. This approach many times is more practical, more efficient, more effective and less costly. Out-service training includes such procedures as visits to other facilities; attendance at professional conferences and meetings; participation in available in-service training programs; and enrollment in home study, adult education, college and university courses.

The availability of training and development opportunities in the local facility or outside it does not assure active and meaningful participation on the part of staff members. Encouragement, direction and even incentives must be made available.

Sometimes it is not enough to circulate a relevant article; it must be followed up by a discussion. Sometimes it is not enough to arrange a visit to another facility; it must involve traveling as a group in a car to "gear up" for a purposeful visit and returning the same way in order to make meaningful application while everyone is ready and eager. Sometimes it is not enough to send someone to a professional conference; he may need guidance concerning sessions to attend and people to seek out. Sometimes it is not enough to request a staff member to attend an adult education or college course; he may need financial assistance, release time or compensatory time.

Like most activities within a rehabilitation facility, personnel training will rise and fall according to the significance the administrator and board of directors give it. Staff training and development's importance comes down from the top of a facility to all the other personnel. Unfortunately, the converse is frequently true resulting in all too familiar personnel training or lack of it.

Consequently, it is imperative that boards of directors' policies and budgets support personnel training as is done in industry and education. It is equally imperative that administrators demonstrate active and positive leadership in making it significant, relevant, continuous and palatable. Without such commitment from the top, the role and contribution of personnel training will be questionable.

Summary

Facilities may be thought of as learning centers for any level of rehabilitation training, and may operate their own programs as well as function as adjuncts to other training programs. In-service training, that which is designed to improve the effectiveness of the individual in the position he now holds, is a need in every facility.

The professional trainer within a facility has several major roles to perform and contributions to make. He is a learning specialist skilled in the ability to use learning theory and methods to meet training needs. He is an information coordinator who seeks, clarifies, synthesizes, reality-tests, and provides information as a communications link within the facility. He is an internal consultant to the facility's administration and management as well as an external consultant to other facilities and organizations. He is an administrator with administrative skills which support his other roles and allow him to function in special assignments. Finally, he is a public relations person because of the exposure the other roles, especially that of learning specialist and consultant, accord him.

Assuming the concepts concerning the traditional distinctions between education and training and between professional and nonprofessional lack credence, in-service training can be designed in three stages: orientation, initial training and ongoing training. The practical procedures covering these stages are numerous and varied. However, only strong support and leadership in personnel training by the administrator and board of directors of the facility will protect personnel training from becoming a periodic intruder. Rather it should be integrated within all of the activities of the facility.

REFERENCES

De Jager, Harvey C.: "The Future of Rehabilitation Personnel Training in Facilities." In *The Role of Facilities in Training Rehabilitation Personnel,* ed. James E. Trela. Cleveland: Vocational Guidance and Rehabilitation Services, 1973, pp. 183–196.

Kozoll, Charles E., and Ulmer, Curtis: *In-Service Training: Philosophy, Proc-*

esses, and Operational Techniques. Englewood Cliffs: Prentice-Hall, 1972, pp. 19–21.

Lippitt, Gordon L.: *Leadership for Learning: Training and Development in the 70's.* American Society for Training and Development. Washington, D. C.: Project Associates, 1970, pp. 18–21.

"Perspective: Harvey C. De Jager." *News and Views, 4,* (2) September–October, 1973, p. 2.

This, Leslie E., and Lippitt, Gordon L.: "Learning Theories and Training —An Overview of Learning Theory Implications for the Training Director." *Training and Development Journal,* 20, (4) April–May, 1966.

Trela, James E. (ed.): *The Role of Facilities in Training Rehabilitation Personnel.* Cleveland: Vocational Guidance and Rehabilitation Services, 1973.

CHAPTER 8

RESEARCH CONSIDERATIONS IN REHABILITATION FACILITIES *

JAMES E. TRELA

☐ Facility Based Research and Researcher Roles

☐ Organizational Impact

☐ Interorganizational Impact

☐ Impact on the Professional Field

PROFESSIONAL SERVICES OF ANY KIND must be supported by two institutionalized activities: the training of personnel in the techniques and norms of practice, and the development of a body of empirically derived and tested knowledge to guide practice. This chapter addresses the latter activity as it is pursued in rehabilitation facilities.

In rehabilitation, and other practice fields, research tends to be identified as something done by university based scientists, and the provision of services is identified as something that is done by facility based practitioners. It is important to note, however, that this division of labor is neither complete nor necessarily appropriate. In fact, research occurs, with varying degrees of frequency and sophistication, in all organizational contexts. In rehabilitation facilities, the need for research based program evaluation is particularly urgent and is becom-

* Parts of this chapter are adapted from Trela and O'Toole, *Roles for Sociologists in Service Organizations* (1974); final report for Social Rehabilitation Service project 12-P-55201.

129

ing more so with the increased emphasis on accountability. This chapter does not deal with the technical aspects of the research enterprise. Rather, its goals are: (1) to briefly discuss the unique nature of facility based research and identify the variety of roles that researchers can play in facilities; and most important, (2) to assess the significance of these roles for both the facility and the field of rehabilitation.

FACILITY BASED RESEARCH AND RESEARCHER ROLES

Research may be defined briefly as the combination of reason and observation directed toward the solution of a problem. While it is not the intent of this chapter to present facility based research as something apart from research conducted in other settings, there are several important distinguishing characteristics.

First, facility based research is predominantly "applied" as opposed to "basic." While many scientists object to this distinction, it is a useful one for roughly differentiating between university and service organization research. The National Science Foundation refers to basic research as "original investigations for the advancement of scientific knowledge" (Vollmer, 1972, p. 67). Such research is not intended to solve the problems or answer the questions of host organizations, although it may be of potential utility to these organizations. Applied research, on the other hand, focuses on problems posed by the host organization and is intended to contribute to the solutions of organizational problems. Research may, of course, have both basic and applied implications, but in most cases a general orientation can be identified. In the case of basic research, it is thought that findings will ultimately benefit society, while in the case of applied research, findings are directed toward the solution of immediate problems. Perhaps the most important kind of applied research for facilities is program evaluation. This is research intended to determine the degree to which organizational activities produce the desired effects. This will be discussed further when we attempt to assess the impact of research on facility operations.

Secondly and more important, in facilities the research enterprise tends to be broadly conceived to encompass a variety of activities which are not research in the strictest sense but which are either research related or capitalize on the researcher's skills. In facilities, or any service setting where a flexible application of skills is often required, this should not be surprising. The term research is highly elastic, not only among practitioners and administrators but among researchers as well. Earning research credentials assumes at least some substantive knowledge of human behavior and social conditions, and some familiarity with programs designed to alter that behavior or ameliorate those conditions. The development of literary skills is also necessary. In a facility, in addition to *research,* related skills are likely to be pressed into service and the researcher may become responsible not only for applied research and program evaluation, but for *program design* as well—especially when the latter involves the preparation of elaborate written requests for funding. Related to these activities, there is a tendency for applied researchers to function in both *administrative* and *liaison* capacities. These roles are natural extensions of the combined research and program design roles. The program designer, for example, is the person most familiar with a project's personnel needs and budget requirements and may be called upon in both the recruitment and orientation of service personnel. Also, some administrative control is necessary for data collection and the preservation of the integrity of research designs. Similarly, dealing with program budget and design, the pursuit of funding, and project problems often involves not only administrative activities, but the initiation and management of interorganizational relationships for the organization. Hence, an important role, which may come to be independent of research activities, is that of liaison with other organizations.

The research, program planning and design, administrative and liaison roles, while perhaps the most important, do not exhaust the roles that a researcher may play in a facility. For example, one of the major requirements of research is the collection, reduction and analysis of data and the communication of subsequent findings. It is natural, then, for *record-keeping* functions to be assigned to the researcher even though most record-keeping systems hold only limited research value. As a consequence, there is a further expansion of the administrative and liaison roles. Not only are staff brought under the supervision of the researcher, but record keeping requires the coordination of data reporters throughout the organization. Similarly, the researcher needs to keep abreast of developments in his discipline and communicate the results of his research to appropriate audiences. These activities blend well with the facility's need to disseminate information about its programs. Hence, the role of *communicator* is differentiated. In this role the researcher is responsible for reviewing and condensing information from the field of rehabilitation (and other disciplines as well) for dissemination to practitioners, and writing about organizational programs and research for dissemination to rehabilitation and other audiences. Information is transmitted to practitioners both through informal channels of communication and formally through project designs, in-service educational programs, and reports to administrators and board members. As with other roles, the communication role may be broadly defined. Because the researcher represents scholarly interests and relies on written material in his communicative role, it follows that he can assist in the collection, preparation and dissemination of materials which are not research related but which concern the facility. Responsibility for the staff library, preparation of annual reports, speeches and testimonies before legislative groups, as well as review of critical communication with other organizations, are examples of such activities.

The role of *educator* is another "natural" role for the researcher to assume in a facility. As a result of his theoretical and methodological training, substantive knowledge in some areas, and teaching skills, a researcher may be requested to contribute to the in-service training of staff as well as formal training programs. Finally, functioning as a resource person within the organization eventually becomes identified as a separate role: that of *consultant* to administrators and practitioners. Hence, several roles for researchers can be identified, including:

RESEARCH: This role consists of designing and initiating research projects including problem formulation, the selection or design of instruments, data collection and processing, data analysis and the preparation of reports and publications. The research may be "basic" or "applied" and may involve collaboration with university colleagues or organizational practitioners.

PROGRAM PLANNING AND DESIGN: In this role the researcher works with administrators, practitioners, and frequently funding agency personnel, to design research and demonstration, service and training projects. This normally includes, in addition to program design, the preparation of budgets and grant applications for outside funding.

ADMINISTRATION: This role includes the supervision of subordinate research workers and consultants, some management of the service component of research projects, and the coordination of research with administrators, service personnel and funding organizations.

LIAISON WITH OTHER ORGANIZATIONS: This role centers on managing interorganizational relations for the agency. Each of the researcher's roles may have an interorganizational component which becomes recognized by other persons as a separate and distinct role. The role consists of initiating and maintaining relationships with other agencies and organizations, responding to requests for client and service data, providing technical resources (as in the preparation of project grants), the disposition of contractual obligations such as final reports, and perhaps negotiating the division of labor in cooperative service ventures.

RECORD KEEPING: In this role the researcher collects, processes, analyzes and communicates data on agency programs and clients. This becomes the basis for both administrative decision making and for reporting activities to funding, accrediting, coordinating and planning organizations at the local, state, and national levels.

COMMUNICATION: In the role of communicator the researcher is at the hub of a network that functions to receive and transmit information for the organization. The researcher, through both informal and formal communication channels, facilitates the reciprocal passage of information between practitioners and administrators, on the one hand, and researchers, practitioners and funders in the field of rehabilitation on the other.

EDUCATION AND TRAINING: Several of the roles performed by the researcher incorporate educational functions including the formal and informal instruction of research assistants and statistical clerks, in-service training of staff and participation in formal rehabilitation training programs.

Organizational Operations

Roles	Areas of Impact
Research	Program Evaluation and Client
Consultation	Follow-up
Program Planning and Design	Program Development
Administration	Staff Effectiveness
Record Keeping	Organizational Development
Communication	Decision Making and Problem
Education and Training	Solving
	Program Accounting

Interorganizational Relations

Roles	Areas of Impact
Liaison	Support and Resources from
Program Planning and Design	Other Organizations
Record Keeping	Accountability and Visability
Communication	

Professional Field Contributions

Roles	Areas of Impact
Research	Linkage of Theory, Research and
Communication	Practice
Education and Training	Production of New Knowledge
Liaison	

Figure 8–1 Research Roles and Areas of Impact

CONSULTATION: In this somewhat residual role the researcher functions as a resource person on specific organizational problems and as a general consultant to administrators and practitioners on organizational planning and program evaluation.

The roles performed by the researcher, of course, are interrelated. Research activities, in a research and development program, for example, may be related to program planning and design and may involve the researcher in liaison and administrative relations within the facility and with outside organizations. Nevertheless, it is possible to identify general outcomes which reflect certain role activities. In Figure 8–1 an attempt is made to specify the relationship between role activities and specific areas of impact at the organizational, interorganizational, and professional field levels of concern. For example, the research role has important consequences for the achievement of organizational and professional goals but has little direct impact on interorganizational relations. Alternatively, the liaison role may have beneficial consequences for interorganizational and professional field goals, but may have little consequence for the organization's internal operations.

Above we identified the array of roles that may be performed by researchers. More important, it is necessary to address the question: does the development of the research role in a facility contribute to the goals of that organization and the larger endeavor of which it is a part? To answer this question, the researcher's roles are analyzed in terms of their impact on: the internal workings of the organization and its programs; the management of the organization's relationships with other organizations; and the organization's contribution to the field of professional practice.

ORGANIZATIONAL IMPACT

Development of the research role in a facility should result in improved program evaluation and client follow-up, more effective program planning and design, increased staff effectiveness, new initiatives in organizational development, more efficient decision making and problem solving and improved internal program accounting. All of these bear directly upon the quality of services facilities provide.

PROGRAM EVALUATION AND CLIENT FOLLOW-UP: The researcher's theoretical and methodological knowledge employed in evaluative research potentially provides the basis for his most significant impact on the internal operations of the facility and its programs. The reason for this, as many have noted, is that one of the greatest needs of all service organizations is for the evaluation of services they provide (Lacks and Plax, 1972). In rehabilitation, for example, the providers of services are often concerned primarily with the process independent of the products of rehabilitation practice. Services are assumed to have beneficial outcomes. It is not uncommon for programs to be judged solely in terms of what is done *for* and *to* clients ("inputs"). The researcher, on the other hand, employing the methods of science, can collect and analyze data and measure the degree to which specified organizational activities produce the desired effects. He focuses on "outcomes" and seeks to determine whether they are the intended results of certain services.

Program evaluation and client follow-up are important in a facility not only because they seek to determine the effectiveness of programs but also because these activities provide the impetus and basis for programmatic change. They also promote a sensitivity to the relationship of means to ends and client benefits to service costs, and encourage exploration for more effective alternative service strategies.

PROGRAM PLANNING AND DESIGN: Closely related to program evaluation is program planning and design. There is a pressing need for those engaged in developing service strategies to be at the frontier of knowledge in their areas of interest. For many good reasons, however, the need is seldom met. In any rapidly changing field, ideas are often ahead of practice and the dissemination and utilization of new ideas and knowledge is always problematic. Research and practice have, in fact, been so detached that information is often outdated before it reaches those who may use it. Equally as important, most research findings never reach the potential user in a form that is easily and directly translated into practice. Recognition of the fact that the communication networks of the "discoverers" and "users" of knowledge are not significantly overlapped has led to repeated calls for a stronger relationship between researcher and practitioner.

The process of program planning and design is strengthened by the researcher's close association with practitioners and his participation in a communication system which helps connect facility personnel to researchers and other practitioners outside the organization. First, through the professional literature and formal and informal associations with professionals outside the facility, the researcher acquires and disseminates new knowledge and procedures within the facility and may be instrumental in insuring the utilization of this knowledge in program planning and design. Just as important, the researcher is in an excellent position to help practitioners translate research knowledge into new strategies for practice. It is this skill that accounts for the tendency for researchers to become involved in program planning and design. Thus, by participating in the professional-scientific communication network, by promoting the linkage of new knowledge with practice, and by drawing out the implications of research for practice, the researcher may have a significant impact on program planning and design and the quality of new facility programs.

STAFF EFFECTIVENESS: It is, of course, apparent that program evaluation contributes directly to the quality of services offered in a facility. Systematic evaluation also has several latent consequences which contribute to quality services. When practitioners realize that the *outcomes* of their efforts are being analyzed and evaluated there are often efforts to improve the quality of services. Also, in completing data reports, practitioners are continually reminded of the goals of service and are provided with the opportunity for periodic self and program evaluation.

The researcher, as an adjunct to his evaluation and program planning roles, may also contribute to practice as a trainer. Rapidly changing organizations are always faced with the problems of training and orienting both new and continuing personnel. This is especially true when innovative programs are being initiated and professional and non-professional personnel must be recruited in a very short time. Researchers, having often designed programs, can help orient staff to program needs and their various roles in a service project. In addition, in his role as educator, the researcher may periodically find it useful to formally remind staff of the goals of the project. Perhaps the major impact of the educational role, however, is informal. Interaction between the researcher and practitioners results in mutual "education." The more effective the researcher is in this interaction, the greater his impact on staff effectiveness and professional practice.

ORGANIZATIONAL DEVELOPMENT: Just as program planning and design are related to the quality of services offered in a facility, it is also related to the direction and rapidity of organizational change and the financial and administrative strength of the organization over time. The researcher, through innovative programming, can be instrumental in securing grant support and other resources for new initiatives.

Often, practitioners, even those with a high level of experience and knowledge, do not feel able to conceptualize, plan, and design a new program and then construct a research design by which it can be evaluated. The researcher's theoretical and substantive knowledge and analytic, methodological and writing skills can be engaged to design new programs and to secure necessary funding for demonstrating projects that expand service offerings and contribute to the development of the facility. For example, the Federal Research and Development grant has been a particularly important vehicle for organizational development. The facility wishing to take advantage of this mechanism must comply with the funder's application, evaluation and reporting requirements. Once the researcher gains experience in program planning and grant writing, these skills can be used for seeking funding for projects of all types. These funds provide for greater organizational flexibility in programming and staffing and afford the opportunity to try out new ideas and patterns of service which would otherwise not be possible. Not incidentally, the facility that is able to develop innovative programs and experiment with its service strategies is most likely to attract the most able staff.

DECISION MAKING AND PROBLEM SOLVING: In addition to placing program planning and development on a more scientific basis, evaluative research is an important aspect of administrative decision making. Indeed, Suchman notes that "evaluative research constitutes the methodological and empirical backbone of any attempt to build a field of administrative science or practice theory" (1971). The evaluative researcher's impact, of course, stems from information he supplies to decision makers and not from his position within the administrative hierarchy. Through consultation, the researcher furnishes information and perhaps recommendations to policy makers and may make additional recommendations with regard to the process of communicating and implementing policy once it had been determined. Information on the efficacy of a particular program or mode of service delivery, of course, is only one element in this process. In addition, scientific knowledge of community structure and minorities can be employed to provide decision makers with alternative perspectives on a problem, and some knowledge about the probable outcomes of administrative decisions.

Closely related to decision making is problem solving. Facilities are often faced with a variety of problems, from devising "short cut" methods of testing a new service strategy to convincing a related service organization to provide services to a given population category. Hence, in addition to using theoretical and substantive knowledge in his field and the interdisciplinary knowledge accumulated in rehabilitation in day-to-day decision making, the researcher can contribute to any problem solving efforts. For example, through his understanding of the structure of organizations and the process by which they function he may be able to show how a problem is due to the structure of the organization and not to the personalities of those involved. Or, the researcher's experience in fields of study other than rehabilitation may provide unexpected analogies and thus broaden the range of alternatives considered by policy makers and practitioners.

In addition to theoretical and substantive knowledge are the researcher's methodological skills. Research is a problem-solving process and hence the researcher should be adept at articulating the important elements of a given problem and designing a procedure for its solution. Hence, any problem-solving process (e.g. the effectiveness of a new case management system) may beneficially include the researcher, even when he lacks relevant substantive expertise.

Perhaps the greatest contribution to organizational problem solving, however, results from the skeptical and critical nature of science. The researcher, having internalized the scientific perspective, is better able to assume a detached posture with regard to policy alternatives. To the degree that he is detached and can legitimize the role of "devil's advocate," the researcher may be able to identify unanticipated consequences of various decisions and suggest more viable alternatives.

PROGRAM ACCOUNTING: One important adjunct to program evaluation and administrative decision making and problem solving is record keeping. There is a great need for the systematic recording of services rendered, numbers and characteristics of clients served, and the other facts related to facility operations. However, service accounting systems utilized in facilities are usually inadequate in a number of ways. They are often not constructed to answer the questions most likely to be asked and therefore cannot produce information for important administrative initiatives. For example, there is a tendency to collect service input information while neglecting service outcome data. Further, they produce data that is often unreliable, under-reported or not comparable for different segments of the organization. Nor do data collection procedures and analysis take advantage of available technologies. These problems are cumulative and result in facility records being an inadequate source of information for administrators and practitioners. In view of these problems, many professionals and service staff give service program accounting low priority compared to other work activities. In turn, there is little utilization of data in program evaluation and decision making.

Faced with the problems of collecting and analyzing large amounts of data, the social and behavioral sciences have adopted or developed techniques for collecting, coding and analyzing data efficiently. Further, these activities can be simplified and accelerated through the use of automatic data processing equipment. In addition, researchers should be adept at drawing out implications of the data in terms of the theoretical or practical administrative problems under consideration.

INTERORGANIZATIONAL IMPACT

Development of the research role in a facility should result in improved interorganizational relations and hence greater ability to secure support or resources from other organizations.

In addition, the facility's ability to establish and maintain a high level of visibility and accountability in its interorganizational environment should be improved.

SUPPORT AND RESOURCES FROM OTHER ORGANIZATIONS: Organizations do not operate in a vacuum and problems are not confined to the relation between the providers and beneficiaries of service. A facility is located in a network of other organizations, some of which are essential not only to its service mission but to its very survival. Also, its relationship with these organizations may alternatively be competitive or cooperative. In a complex field such as rehabilitation, in which private organizations and public agencies at all levels of government are interrelated, a great deal of energy can be devoted to establishing and maintaining interorganizational relationships. For example, on its own, a facility may act as a training center for the staff of other organizations; a research setting for a university based study; and a service setting for the clients of other organizations. Similarly, on its own a facility may seek funding or other kinds of support from a variety of organizations; advocate client interests with other organizations; share in the division of labor for providing services to a given client population; and provide consultation and information for area, regional and national coordinating and planning agencies.

In many of the roles the researcher plays he must establish and maintain relationships with a number of organizations on behalf of the facility's interests. Many of these relationships increase the facility's competitiveness in the struggle for scarce resources. This is not surprising. These relationships, both formal and informal, provide channels for communication and hence become sources of information and means for influencing the activities of other organizations. Knowledge about the interests and priorities of other key organizations as well as appropriate procedures for relating to these organizations is especially critical. Without this knowledge it is extraordinarily difficult to develop cooperative programs, coordinate services or secure funds.

This may be illustrated by the Research and Development

grant, which often requires relationships with both public and private organizations. In order to secure an R and D grant, a facility must often present its program to state, regional and national levels of a funding agency. Similarly, the promise of the program may be contingent upon both mobilizing various kinds of expertise and coordinating activities with other community organizations. Hence, relations may have to be established with a nearby university and service may have to be coordinated with various referring organizations in the community. It may also be necessary to secure approval from neighborhood and other citizen, client, and political groups. Through the channels of communications he establishes with other organizations, the researcher can determine which organizations will be most likely to fund a given program, identify the best way to present ideas and develop the grant package, determine the details and procedures necessary for submitting application, develop mechanisms for coordinating services with other key organizations, and secure approval and support from appropriate publics. These activities not only increase the probability that a given program will be approved for funding but that it will be accepted by referring organizations, client groups and others who may believe that their interests are either furthered or compromised by its implementation.

ACCOUNTING AND VISIBILITY: Facilities are accountable to a number of publics and decision-making bodies. These may include its own board of directors, the client community, client referring agencies, several funding agencies, coordinating and accrediting bodies and the community in which the facility is located. While it remains true that humanitarian goals are often offered as a justification for a program's existence in general, the social service field has moved toward accountability based upon systematic assessment of psychological, social and economic outcomes. Further, the ability of an organization to "give a good accounting of itself" has become increasingly important as resources have become scarce, competition for those that exist has become more fierce, and public confidence in the ability of the helping professions has deteriorated.

Public and decision-making bodies ask: "What proof is there that a program works?" "How much does it cost?" and "Is it worth the cost?" Hence, administrators are increasingly faced with the task of having to supply data that essentially divides the total cost of a program by the number of successful client outcomes.

These changes in the demands made upon a facility have greatly increased the need for evaluation and the analysis and presentation of records according to more scientific standards. These are activities which call for research-related knowledge and skills. The researcher can contribute to and demonstrate the setting's effectiveness to those whose resources and cooperation are required by: quantifying what is being done, measuring program outcomes by documenting whether or not change has occurred as a result of rendered services, and developing measures of the relationship between client benefits and program service costs. This contributes to the confidence other organizations have in the facility and its programs and insures support and additional resources for growth.

A closely related aspect of the researcher's roles relates to increased visibility of the facility and its programs to various publics. While it may be true that "good work is all that matters," it is also true that a facility's public image and relations are important if it is to be used by clients and attract good personnel and support (e.g. board members, grants, etc.). While public relations is somewhat outside the interests of the researcher, in several ways he can be instrumental in increasing the visibility and enhancing the image of the facility, especially at the national and professional levels.

First, one benefit of having a research position in a service organization is that it enhances the organization's prestige vis-á-vis other similar organizations. This is especially true in rehabilitation facilities, few of which have a strong tradition of research.

Second, and more important, increasing the visibility of the agency is a product directly or indirectly of the research enterprise. The image of the facility as well as specific knowledge concerning its activities must be communicated to organizations and persons who are in a position to lend support. The researcher's publications, reports, and conference papers describe the facility's programs and this, in turn, helps justify its claim to high standards of professional practice. It may be added that visibility also has important consequences for internal facility operations insofar as it increases morale and staff commitment to the organization and its goals.

IMPACT ON THE PROFESSIONAL FIELD

The essential rationale for establishing a research role in a rehabilitation facility or any service organization is to improve the effectiveness of programs and the quality of service. Previous sections have shown how the researcher in various roles can contribute to these goals within the facility and its interorganizational environment. Equally as important, the facility based researcher can contribute to the goals of the rehabilitation field by narrowing the gap between practice and both theory and research and contributing to the body of knowledge that supports rehabilitation practice.

NARROWING THE GAP BETWEEN PRACTICE, THEORY AND RESEARCH: The gap between theory and research, on the one hand, and practice, on the other, seems to be forever with us. Referring to the estrangement of theory and practice, Galileo declared that those who like to theorize about nature ought to go into the shops and shipyards and watch artisans and mechanics at work. Similarly, in rehabilitation, those who theorize and do research about human behavior and institutions seem to be detached from those who work with people. This is hardly surprising in view of the separation and concentration of researchers and trainers in university settings and practitioners in service settings. Nor is this separation purely organizational. More important, the individuals who work in these settings are differentiated by the values they share and the norms that govern their behavior.

Of course, the thought that practitioners might contribute in university and college settings and researchers might contribute in service settings is not new or untried. It has, however, failed to be institutionalized sufficiently to ensure the union of research, theory and practice. Hence, the facility based researcher, because of his close proximity to practice, is in a position to ensure that research is grounded in the world to which it is intended to contribute. He can do this in two ways: by tailoring his own research to the needs of the practitioner and by translating practitioner interests and problems into research ideas and problems for rehabilitation and related disciplines.

Just as researchers and theorists have been detached from practitioners, the latter often seem oblivious to the source of knowledge and ideas that form the basis for practice. Practitioners utilize theoretical formulations to make hypotheses about the nature and etiology of disabilities and the type of intervention needed to produce desired change. These theoretical notions guiding practice, however, quite often are implicit, unsystematic and unorganized. This makes it difficult to recognize inconsistencies and select key elements to improve upon or test. It is also largely impossible to adapt such crude formulatons to other organizational and community settings.

One important contribution of the social scientist in the field of rehabilitation may be to help provide theoretical frameworks which organize the important factors in the rehabilitation process. In this process one of the important aspects of the role of the researcher is to "follow" and observe practitioners in the rehabilitation situation. His goal is to provide theories which explain the relationship between intervention of a particular type and rehabilitation outcomes. He utilizes theories from the social and behavioral sciences to help tease out those factors which seem to be critical to the process of change as well as those which provide the context for the process. Once ideas are stated in a theoretical manner they can be tested and rejected or modified. Theories may point to contradictions or suggest new insights for practice by pointing to logical extensions of practice techniques or procedures. The contribution of the researcher to the integration of practice, theory and research, then, is twofold: the researcher links research and theory to the world of practice; and provides theory which allows practitioners to organize practice and see the relationship between critical variables in the rehabilitation process.

CONTRIBUTIONS TO KNOWLEDGE: It was noted earlier that the researcher functions as a communication link between practitioners, the practice field and related scientific disciplines. As a receiver and interpreter of information the researcher can promote the utilization of new knowledge and have a major impact on the internal functioning of the organization and its programs. Equally as significant, the researcher can provide the facility with an opportunity to contribute significantly to knowledge not only in the area of rehabilitation practice but to scientific knowledge in psychology, sociology, and other related disciplines as well. This can be done both through the dissemination of research results and program evaluation findings produced within the facility and the use of the facility to test and demonstrate new programs. The facility with research capabilities is a particularly appropriate environment for testing new ideas and innovative programs as well as doing more basic research on the dynamics of human behavior.

The linking of information utilization and dissemination roles in one organizational position, that of facility researcher, may provide one solution to the dissemination-utilization problems which plague fields of practice and their related scientific disciplines. It is in facilities where new programs must be tested and where the everyday practice of rehabilitation comes to life. In publications and in the presentation of papers at professional meetings, applied research results on facility programs can be communicated to a wide audience of rehabilitation personnel. Further, the researcher can collaborate with facility personnel, and by contributing his conceptual, organizational, and writing skills, can promote practitioner-oriented publications. In this manner, practitioner knowledge and problems are communicated to professionals and researchers, and practitioner interests are translated into problems that are relevant to researchers. The researcher's position as a communication link between research and practice serves both the facility and the field of rehabilitation. Information is brought into the facility to be utilized in program design and evaluative research and other research findings are communicated through these same channels to practitioners and researchers in other settings.

SUMMARY

This chapter has attempted to demonstrate that there are many roles that researchers may play in a rehabilitation facility. In addition to conducting both basic and applied research, including program evaluation, the researcher may function in the areas of program planning and design, administration, liaison with other organizations, record keeping, communication, education, and consultation. The impact of these various roles may be seen at three levels. At the organizational level the researcher may contribute to improved program evaluation, more effective program planning and design, increased staff effectiveness, new initiatives in organizational development, more efficient decision making and problem solving and improved internal program accounting. At the interorganizational level the researcher may contribute to improved and more effective relations with other organizations, thereby increasing the ability of the facility to secure support and cooperation. The researcher may also increase the facility's visibility and accountability with its various publics. Finally, the researcher can contribute to the professional field by helping narrow the gap between practice and research and by adding to the body of knowledge that supports practice.

REFERENCES

Lacks, P.B., and Plax, K.A.: *A Research Program for a Vocational Rehabilitation Agency.* St. Louis: Jewish Employment and Vocational Service, May, 1972.

Suchman, E.: "Action for What: A Critique of Evaluation Research." In R. O'Toole, *The Organization, Management, and Tactics of Social Research.* Cambridge: Schenkman Publishing, 1971, pp. 97–130.

Trela, J.E., and O'Toole, R.: *Roles for Sociologists in Service Organizations.* Kent: The Kent State University Press, 1974.

Vollmer, M.V.: "Basic and Applied Research" in S.Z. Nagi and R.G. Corwin, *The Social Context of Research.* New York: Wiley-Interscience, 1972, 67–96.

CHAPTER 9

CONSIDERATIONS OF STATE VOCATIONAL REHABILITATION AGENCY RELATIONSHIPS

NATHAN B. NOLAN

☐ Purchase of Services

☐ Facilities Specialists

☐ Accreditation and Standards

☐ Community Involvement

IN ORDER TO VIEW a relationship between two organizations it is often helpful to review the goals and missions of those organizations. While rehabilitation facilities generally concern themselves with the provision of specific types of service, often to a specific type or group of people and to a relatively limited geographical area, the state agency must be more global in its approach since it is charged with the responsibility of dealing with at least an entire state and with all groups of handicapped or disabled people. The agency, therefore, is in a position to provide leadership in overall planning for a large geographical area and to work with individual facilities in fitting their particular services into an overall plan for many additional people. It is usually charged by various official groups with certain responsibilities for planning, directing, projecting, predicting, and generally providing leadership in the area of growth and development of the rehabilitation movement.

148

The rehabilitation agency receives its "charter" from the body politic and is held accountable to this body. It therefore sees itself as an official type representative of the entire citizenry of the state, and of the state itself, in the area of rehabilitation and service to disabled people. It has some responsibility to the citizenry to avoid unnecessary duplication of services and to insure that rehabilitation services are efficiently and effectively provided.

The state rehabilitation agency receives its funding almost entirely from tax sources. It is therefore governed by laws and regulations which surround the provision of funds, both state and federal. The central goal of the rehabilitation agency is "to return" disabled individuals to remunerative employment. Interpretation has broadened the word "return" to include helping individuals to enter employment and the word "remunerative" has been broadened to include unpaid family workers and homemakers. Some state agencies also include in this definition employment which is less than self-sustaining and thus consider sheltered employment in workshops as an appropriate vocational goal. It should be noted, however, that the definitions include only the provision of services which are designed to move an individual toward employment. Also inherent in the program is a time factor which requires that results be obtained in a "reasonable" period of time.

As one works with social programs which are the result of Federal and State legislation, one must be constantly aware of changing emphasis, of financing, and other vital factors which affect the programs. Society, by shifting its emphasis, its support, and by an ever-changing approach to meet demands which have not been fully met, constantly challenges people who feel they have developed a sound appropriate approach to make changes in those approaches.

One of the characteristics of state vocational rehabilitation agencies has been the incorporation of new ideas and practices in the provision of services to its clients. During the 1960's, nothing had been more significant than the growing use of, and dependence upon, rehabilitation facilities to serve severely handicapped vocational rehabilitation clients. As might be expected, issues have arisen from time to time. These issues have developed around such questions as who the rehabilitation agency should send to the facility for service, what control the agency should maintain over the individual's "rehabilitation plan," how much rehabilitation facility services of various kinds should cost, methods of payment for services that are most satisfactory to both the facility and the rehabilitation agency, and how to assure quality control of services.

Several systems of cooperative arrangements with governmental and non-governmental institutions serving handicapped people have been developed in recent years. The Council of State Administrators of Vocational Rehabilitation, an organization of top administrators of the various state agencies, adopted a statement in May, 1972, which set a pattern for relationships between rehabilitation facilities and vocational rehabilitation agencies.[1]

The Council summarizes the functions of State Vocational Rehabilitation Agencies as follows:

1. The evaluation of disabled and other disadvantaged individuals and the provision of comprehensive vocational rehabilitation services to those eligible under rehabilitation legislation.
2. Continuous statewide planning directed toward current assessments of the needs of handicapped individuals and how these needs can be most effectively met.
3. Exercising leadership in the development of facilities and programs needed in the rehabilitation of the handicapped.
4. Developing and maintaining cooperative relationships and programs with public and private agencies in the state and its communities.
5. Performing functions related to federal acts in addition to the Vocational Rehabilitation Act, such as providing minor medical services for persons served under the Manpower Development and Training Act, making disability determinations for the Social Security Administration, and making certifications to the Department of Labor under the Fair Labor Standards Act with respect to certain activities in workshops and as to the earning capacity of handicapped individuals who have completed training or evaluation programs.

[1] Guidelines for Working Relationships Between VR Agencies and Rehabilitation Facilities—Council of State Administrators of Vocational Rehabilitation.

6. Exercising leadership in research and in the training of individuals who are to serve handicapped individuals.

It should be noted that the role of the vocational rehabilitation agency has both service and leadership components.

It is obvious that state rehabilitation agencies are making more and more use of rehabilitation facilities. This is demonstrated in the increasing expenditures by these agencies for services in rehabilitation facilities and in the increasing number of handicapped individuals who are being sent to these facilities for services. The role of the rehabilitation facility is described by this Council as follows:

1. In numerous cases, the rehabilitation facility is needed to assist the vocational rehabilitation agency in determining the rehabilitation potential of the individual, with special emphasis on his work potential.
2. Rehabilitation facilities are needed to provide vocational training and adjustment services for many vocational rehabilitation clients.
3. The facility is needed to assist in making determinations of disability for many individuals making application for old age and survivors disability benefits and, as already indicated, to provide similar services for applicants for welfare benefits.
4. The facility constitutes a laboratory in which research into the problems and needs of handicapped individuals may be conducted, and the rehabilitation facility may, itself, conduct pertinent research of value to vocational rehabilitation agencies.
5. Likewise, the rehabilitation facility constitutes an admirable laboratory for the training of staff, not only for working in rehabilitation facilities but for working in vocational rehabilitation and related agencies.
6. The rehabilitation facility can share with the state rehabilitation agency the role of advocacy for the handicapped individual.
7. Since it provides a place where one can see handicapped people actually undergoing the process of rehabilitation, it can acquaint the community with the needs of the handicapped, what is being done to help them, and how the needs may be more effectively met.

The rehabilitation facility is especially valuable in the provision of various services to the very seriously disabled. Here, in a controlled environment, a group of professional people can apply their skills in a coordinated way directed toward the peculiar needs of the particular individual. More than likely, this activity resembles that of competitive and productive work and is designed to either move the individual toward competitive productive work or to provide productive activity for him. Coupled with this are many other services usually provided to enhance the central activity and goal.

As society recognizes more and more the benefits of full utilization of individual potential, as modern medicine continues to develop and sustain life for more and more seriously impaired individuals, and as rehabilitation science develops the ability to understand and predict individual potential, a maximum utilization of rehabilitation resources and techniques becomes imperative. Society's ability to effectively rehabilitate some of its most seriously impaired and disabled individuals can be vastly enhanced through a continued expanding effective partnership between rehabilitation agencies and rehabilitation facilities. Effective partnerships are developed and maintained because each partner has a peculiar and significant contribution to make and because each partner gains something of value from the relationship. They can be maintained only as long as the partners show mutual respect for each other.

In the agency-facility partnership, it is highly desirable, perhaps essential, that the facility reasonably understand the goals, objectives, and points of view of the agency; likewise, the agency needs to understand these things about the facility and it is imperative, if the partnership is to be effective, that mutual respect be maintained. While respect must be earned and continually reinforced, a recognition of the essentiality of this mutual characteristic in a partnership can do much to cement relationships.

PURCHASE OF SERVICES

Traditionally, vocational rehabilitation agencies have purchased services for their clients on a "fee-for-service" basis. The rehabilitation agency has a multitude of dealings with established providers of services, such as colleges, vocational schools, hospitals, physicians, psychologists, and artificial appliance companies of various types. These represent long-established business types which have accepted methods of operation including financing and sale of services. They generally sell to many purchasers and the vocational rehabilitation agency may purchase a large or small amount of the total services offered. Obviously, the relationship with the rehabilitation facility is quite different. The facility is a new phenomenon and does not have an established and well-understood method of selling its services. Its finances often are not tied directly to its provision of services. More often than not, it has been established to provide needed services not elsewhere available and more often than not, those who need the services cannot pay for them.

The rehabilitation agency is often the primary, if not the only purchaser of services from the rehabilitation facility. The relationship is complicated by the fact that many vocational rehabilitation agencies do not have an even flow of available funds with which to purchase services. The facility sometimes refers to this relationship as one of "feast or famine." Through the years, a few principles related to the purchase of services from facilities by state agencies have evolved which the State Council of Rehabilitation Agencies has adopted. It should be recognized that in this listing there are wide variances between state agencies in the application of these principles or, for that matter, even the acceptance of the principles.

The Council recommends that: [2]

1. The state agency should accept responsibility for all reasonable cost associated with serving its clients in rehabilitation facilities. This means that the agency will pay on a "cost" basis for the services its clients receive.
2. The state agency must insist on paying only the cost for those services its clients receive. For instance, if a facility provides medical services and vocational services, and the agency is purchasing only vocational services, it cannot be expected to pay the total "per diem" cost of all rehabilitation services provided in the facility. The accounting system of the facility must be able to cost out the specific services which are being purchased by the vocational rehabilitation agency. Fortunately, accounting systems are now available

[2] Ibid.

which, if adopted by rehabilitation facilities, make this kind of cost accounting practical.

3. The rehabilitation agency must recognize that a rehabilitation facility cannot serve rehabilitation clients effectively unless it can have reasonable assurance at the beginning of the year with respect to the volume of agency clients it will serve during the year. The "feast or famine" method of purchasing services is demoralizing to the rehabilitation facility and not conducive to the long range best interests of rehabilitation agency clients.

4. Rehabilitation agencies cannot operate on the basis that they will purchase services where they are cheapest; neither is it wholesome for rehabilitation facilities to be put in a position of competing for the state agency dollar. State agencies must evaluate carefully the scope and nature of the services they receive from each facility, and agree upon a rate which is fair and reasonable, taking into consideration all aspects of the rehabilitation facility's program and operation. For instance, sometimes it may be to an agency's advantage to pay a high cost to a rehabilitation facility during the year it is becoming established in a community. Later, when its operation has been stabilized, the agency would probably expect the cost of services in such a facility to approximate the cost in long-established facilities.

5. It is the obligation of both the state vocational rehabilitation agency and the rehabilitation facility to work out carefully plans for the evaluation of services provided vocational rehabilitation clients. This is an important but difficult field in which research is badly needed.

In developing relationships with state agencies, the rehabilitation facility needs to develop a plan that will insure an orderly flow of clients and therefore an orderly flow of income from the state agency. This should enable the facility to do intelligent planning in terms of its staff, purchase of supplies, etc. In order to do this, the facility will need to be careful to work closely with the state agency in assessing the needs of the rehabilitation clients and developing a program to meet those needs. It needs to be careful to arrange its charges to the vocational rehabilitation agency to receive adequate compensation for the services provided but carefully avoid the appearance of making a profit on the services. It should be especially careful to move rehabilitation agency clients expeditiously toward a vocational objective and toward employment. Every effort should be made to move a client from the facility into employment as soon as the client is ready for such employment. It is incumbent upon the facility, if it is to maintain good working relationships with rehabilitation agencies, that it provide some kind of effective employment assistance.

Many of the problems between facilities and agencies have revolved around the sensitive pocketbook nerve. Money seems to fairly quickly become an emotional matter. Several reasonably acceptable methods of arriving at a proper financial arrangement between these two parties have been worked out over the years. Various states have devised methods which have worked. Descriptive names for these methods have also been devised. Among these are block funding, contract, purchase of services, and level of payment agreement. These have varied from state to state depending somewhat on the particular point of view prevailing at the moment and the immediate need confronting the state agency with regard to its relationship with facilities. These methods often attract the attention of state officials outside the state rehabilitation agency and thus need to be well defined and relatively easily understood. They all require individual modification and careful application to local situations.

Some state agencies have been able to establish various levels of services provided in rehabilitation facilities, describing rather objectively the characteristics of various levels of services. These sometimes include a listing of types of services; such as psychological services, vocational evaluation services, assessment services, training services, and the like. They sometimes include the level of professional qualifications of staff, prescribing certain academic and experience levels; they sometimes include a listing of related services provided such as social work, counseling, religious activities, etc. These then are divided into groups and a fee is assigned for each level of service. This method places a facility in a good position to use initiative and innovation to effect good programs at minimum cost and thus obtain for itself the benefits of its own effectiveness. It has some disadvantages in that it does not recognize directly the cost of providing rehabilitation services from one setting to another and at times the facility is forced to either abandon a service or to provide it for a fee which represents considerably less than cost. Upgrading and improving services are not easily financed under this method. This system also seems to be conducive to overpaying some facilities while underpaying others.

Another method is based upon the cost accounting principle. The rehabilitation agency describes the service it would like to purchase for its clients from the facility and the number of clients it expects to refer. The facility then prepares a budget which will enable it to finance these services to these clients. The agency agrees to meet this budget through some kind of convenient arrangement that accommodates the accounting systems of the facility and of the agency. Some system of accounting for cost incurred and of revising payments to conform to actual cost is essential. This provides the facility with a reasonably assured steady income over the agreed period and assures the facility of recovering the cost of providing the services. It does not reward the facility for its own efficiency in operation and can be conducive to lackadaisical management and may stifle initiative and innovative approaches. It enables the agency to purchase an appropriate amount of service and assure for itself and its clients the availability of this service on a continuing basis. It appears to be entirely fair to both parties concerned.

A step-by-step process taken from one state program illustrates some of the practical approaches to this method:

Phase I—The state agency develops a list of the amount and type of service purchased from each workshop during the preceding 12 months.

Phase II—The local administrators and supervisors of the state agency and the facilities specialist evaluate the pattern of purchasing service over the period of 12 months.

PHase III—The workshops are contacted by the facilities specialist and the local agency office and requested to make financial records and caseload statistics available for review in developing approximate costs for the provision of rehabilitation services.

Phase IV—A meeting of workshop administrators, workshop counseling staff, state field office administrators and supervisors, a representative group of rehabilitation counselors, "the purchasing agents", as well as the facilities specialist, is scheduled. This meeting allows the local field office staff to project, on the basis of last year's experience and other relevant data, the amount and type of service that will be needed during the following year. The workshop staff describes the types and numbers of personnel, materials and equipment and other factors they believe will be necessary to provide the services requested by the state field office staff. Information obtained by the facilities specialist earlier makes it possible to develop a budget for the level of service proposed. This procedure gives the local field office staff of the state agency a chance to adjust the level of service and the cost of providing the service through mutual negotiation with the workshop staff. A formalized contract between the state agency and each workshop for the support of professional rehabilitation workshop programs of a quality capable of providing a specified amount of service is then entered into. This results in the availability of workshop services to clients of the state agency at a cost which the field counselors feel is compatible with the overall program. It also assures the administrator of the workshop that the cost of maintaining services requested by the state agency would be reimbursed at a predetermined level on a monthly basis for a specific period. There is also a built-in requirement for communication planning and agreement between state agency staff and the workshop staff.

Phase V—The workshop is required to submit claims for reimbursement under a line item budget. Departure from such a budget requires approval of the agency.

Phase VI—At the end of ten months of a one-year contract, the state agency staff and the workshop staff convene a meeting to review and evaluate the results of the contract. A new contract for continuation is drawn up if it is found that the basic agreement is of practical value to all parties. Sufficient evaluation is built into the contract during the year to permit joint development of changes when found to be necessary.

State vocational rehabilitation agencies have become large purchasers of facility services over the years. By 1970, nearly one third of the case service budgets of the state agencies is spent on facility services. Basically, the state agency is looking for the following advantages in formalizing one of the aforementioned types of agreement with a facility:

1. Availability of needed services
2. Input into the clients' programs of services
3. Quality control monitoring of facility services

4. Method of cost review
5. Development of new programs

The rehabilitation facility, on the other hand, may view this kind of arrangement as advantageous in that it allows:

1. Provision of additional resources for client services
2. Provision of additional resources for improvement and expansion of services.

Both groups are desirous of developing a system for arriving at a joint agreement which advances their common interests and which gives each a degree of both freedom and control.

FACILITIES SPECIALISTS

One of the primary responsibilities of state rehabilitation agencies is to continually devise improved methods for meeting the needs of the handicapped individuals it serves. More and more, it is learning that by including a heavy emphasis on the use of rehabilitation facilities, new and improved techniques to rehabilitation are developed. The agency is devoting more and more of its staff time to the developing, nurturing, monitoring, supervising, and generally upgrading the use of rehabilitation facilities. The agency has considerable responsiblity to provide planning which would establish in priority terms the need for additional facilities at various geographical locations as well as the need for additional facilities to provide specific types of services. It obviously must involve many other planning groups and the community generally in these considerations and determinations.

Most state agencies have developed an administrative unit within their organization devoted to these activities. As a result of this activity, the state agency has available a wealth of information that gives up-to-date specifics about the development of new services, new techniques, and the availability of professional training opportunities. Effective relationships between facilities and agencies make this kind of information available to the facility.

This facility unit generally is charged with the responsibility of upgrading the agency use of facilities, of informing and influencing the agency's counselors about facilities and how they should be used. This unit should act as an effective liaison between the independent facility and the state agency counselor.

It is advantageous for staff of the facility unit of the state agency and staff of independent facilities to belong to the same professional organizations, to attend joint training conferences, and generally perform in a way that indicates that they accept a common professional discipline and objective.

ACCREDITATION AND STANDARDS

It is obvious that any purchaser of services is interested in the quality of services it purchases. Accrediting groups for medical services, including both hospitals' and physicians' services, educational and training services have long been used. However, in these instances, as with a determination of fees for services, other large groups of purchasers have also been interested in the standardization, accreditation, and certification. Therefore, the rehabilitation agencies have more or less followed suit with the established measurements of quality within the field affected. The rehabilitation facility is so new that established measures of quality are still in the developmental stages. Most rehabilitation agencies have established some standards of their own; some of these very sophisticated and precise, some very general and simple. They do, however, represent a recognition of the necessity for such standards and a beginning effort to decide what is appropriate.

More recently, several national organizations dedicated to the accreditation of rehabilitation facilities have arisen and the Council of State Administrators of Vocational Rehabilitation has stated that it strongly supports the concept that accreditation by a voluntary agency set up specifically for accreditation purposes. It favors accreditation bodies which operate independently of the institutions they accredit. This is entirely consistent with the state agency's approach in other areas where it purchases services. Many state agencies, however, are extremely guarded as they consider the adoption of a "requirement" that a facility be accredited before the state agency purchases services from it.

The state agencies, generally, want the ability to innovate, expand, and experiment in terms of facility services and want to guard against any hampering of this by an outside agency. A pattern which has developed in the area of hospitalization may well be the one which will develop with facilities. Some state agencies require that hospitals be accredited by the Joint Council on Accreditation of Hospitals; others require that those not accredited by this Council meet certain standards established by the state agency. There is no general requirement throughout the nation that any particular standard of hospital services be provided before rehabilitation agencies authorize purchase of services from them.

Several national groups meet these prerequisites and are providing accreditation to facilities; often with the complete cooperation of the state agency. This accreditation also is having some effect upon other purchasers of services, such as insurance companies providing coverage for workmen's compensation accidents, automobile accidents, etc. It is entirely possible that in future years this will have a marked effect upon the provision of services under systems of national health insurance.

In many instances, state agencies will insist upon on-site monitoring of services in rehabilitation facilities. This type of monitoring is not foreign to rehabilitation agencies in its system of purchase of services although in many instances it does purchase services without monitoring; however, these are usually from long-established vendors. If a facility expects to sell services to a rehabilitation agency in a volume which will have significant effect upon its budget, it needs to accept an on-site monitoring by the rehabilitation agency. It will be extremely helpful to the facility if it can determine in very precise terms what the agency intends to monitor and how it intends to measure its own requirements.

COMMUNITY INVOLVEMENT

Many facilities throughout the country have found it advantageous to include members of the state vocational rehabilitation agency staff on their boards of control. There is a debatable point of ethics involved when this is done since sometimes a conflict of interest arises between a provider of services and a purchaser of services. This procedure, however, is quite often used in a great many other fields, including the private sector. It is necessary that boards of control, if they are to be effective, be composed of people who have enough knowledge about what is to be controlled to effectively and efficiently exert judgment. Bankers serve on boards of directors of facilities who deposit money in their banks. This same principle is true with regard to lawyers, doctors, ministers, and many other professional disciplines. It perhaps is the same in the vocational rehabilitation agencies.

As a matter of practical experience, many facilities throughout the country, have cemented relationships with rehabilitation agencies by placing appropriate members of the agency's staff on their boards. The agency very often has seen the facility in a different light when members of their staff are charged with some responsibility for directing the operations of the facility. The joint involvement of the agency staff, the facility staff, and the community in general in planning processes seems to more effectively determine needs and establish desired goals and, at the same time, helps to insure that these needs and goals will be met through a merging of available resources in the community.

CHAPTER 10

CONSIDERATIONS FOR THE EFFECTIVE UTILIZATION OF CONSULTATION

JOHN G. CULL AND RICHARD E. HARDY

☐ Introduction

☐ Constitution and Bylaws

☐ Public Relations

☐ Advisory Committees

☐ Referral Systems

☐ Case Recording Systems

☐ Needs of Clients

☐ Staff Development Programs

☐ Assessment of Safety in the Rehabilitation Facility

☐ Modification of Jobs and Work Stations

INTRODUCTION

CONSULTATION IS ONE OF MANY necessary ingredients to good rehabilitation facility development and operations. The rehabilitation profession is growing in size and complexity at such a pace it is not possible for any one administrator to be able to keep pace with all the developments. Therefore, he should have at his disposal high quality consultative services. While we feel ongoing consultative services are necessary for viable growth and professionalism in rehabilitation facilities the rehabilitation facility administrator will at times find short-

162

term intensive consultation essential. If the administrators are not familiar with using professional consultants when the time comes to employ them for short periods they generally do not know how to use consultants for deriving maximum effectiveness. In this chapter we will outline a few of the ways in which consultants can be of value to the program and the administrator of the facility.

With the passage of Public Law 89–333 in 1965, the Technical Assistance Program for Workshops and Rehabilitation Centers was established. Technical assistance is authorized by Section 13 (C) of the Vocational Rehabilitation Amendments. The consultation, which is free of cost to the workshop or facility, is provided in areas such as the provision of medical, psychological, social, vocational and other rehabilitation services within facilities; the utilization of subprofessional and support personnel in rehabilitation facilities; vocational evaluation and work adjustment techniques and practices; plant layout, contract procurement, wage standards, industrial engineering assistance, accounting, planning for efficient production on new contracts, work simplification, labor relations, quality control. The rehabilitation facility or workshop receives this consultation merely by requesting it through the State Vocational Rehabilitation Agency. This provision for short-term intensive consultation has been provided for also in the new Rehabilitation Act of 1973.

CONSTITUTION AND BYLAWS

All private or public fund profit corporations established for rehabilitation purposes have a constitution or bylaws which stipulate goals of the facility and the manner in which the facility will achieve those goals. Often the constitution does not facilitate the function of the facility as it should. The constitution should provide broad principals which may be translated into operations; however, the constitution of an organization can become so restrictive that it impedes the progress of the facility and diminishes the value of services provided. Conversely the constitution may be written so loosely and stated in such brief and all-encompassing terms that it provides little if any structure for the board and the facility and few if any guidelines for the operational staff.

Repeatedly we have found that an ill-conceived and poorly articulated constitution is the basis for operational problems in a facility. When a rehabilitation facility staff and its board attempt to diagnose problems in the facility operations, they rarely start at a level as basic as the constitution.

A valid role of a consultant is the evaluation of the bylaws followed by consultation with the board and the operations staff. The consultant may then wish to make specific recommendations for amending the constitution or perhaps totally rewriting it.

PUBLIC RELATIONS

Perhaps the most valuable asset a facility has is a positive public image. If it is positive it is to be revered and protected. If the public image is negative, work on changing it should take precedence over all else. These are strong value judgments; however, the public's view of the facility has a direct and immediate bearing on the quality of services to clients and the future of service programs. Often it is quite difficult for those most closely involved with the facility's operations to be effective in assessing the public image of the program and in determining the public's support for the program, which in turn eventually determines public financial support of the program. By the time the public expresses its lack of support by reducing or cutting off funding support, so much damage has been done to the public's image that it is an uphill battle to restore the faith and confidence of the community.

We have found many causes for lack of support—personality conflicts, a poorly informed public, a deteriorating service program, etc. However, it is of prime importance to assess public support in terms of the public image of the facility prior to obvious trouble if the much-needed support of the program is to continue smoothly. The technical consultant should be used in a constructive manner which will assist in the program operations and not in diagnosing the sources of obvious difficulties. The consultant can fill a valid need in this latter case; however, it is a better administrative technique to call him in earlier than wait until trouble reaches epidemic proportions.

The public image of a facility consists of attitudes relating to purposes of the facility, its location, staff, funding, and clientele. The public image is influenced by attitudes of the staff and their image in the community. It is important to assess public opinion; an outside consultant can help.

ADVISORY COMMITTEES

The Advisory Committee or Advisory Board of a facility should not be confused with the Board of Directors of the facility. The Advisory Board has no administrative or policy-making role. It is concerned exclusively with advising the director and staff of the facility. The Advisory Board may be appointed officially, but it has no officially stipulated duties other than the providing of advice and council.

The Advisory Committee should be a valuable asset which provides good council to the administrator. At times this committee can become so powerful that it "outshines" the Board of Directors. In this situation the Advisory Committee has been allowed to usurp power. We must also guard against the inactive Advisory Committee. If it is inactive, a valuable asset is wasted. The consultant can help the facility achieve a productive balance between these two extremes.

REFERRAL SYSTEMS

Referrals are the lifeblood of the facility. If the referrals are too few, inappropriate, or unduly grouped over a short time span, the facility will experience difficulties in maintaining a viable service program. Perhaps the first step in evaluating the overall referral system is to evaluate the existing referrals and actual clientele of the facility. This evaluation is in relation to the stated purpose and objectives of the facility, the service programs of the facility, and the staff (this latter aspect of the referral system evaluation includes the professional staffing pattern, the supportive staffing pattern, and the number and level of training staff, and the goals and client objectives which the staff wishes to achieve). If the staff of the facility has a strong sense of professionalism and keenly feels a sense of specificity of service, but, in order to maintain a financial viability, the administration accepts all referrals regardless of the needs of the client or the ability of the facility to serve the client, the facility has a severe problem with its development of an adequate referral system.

The second step in evaluating the referral system is to look at the system itself: What are the primary and secondary sources of referral? To answer this compound question the consultant should develop a frequency distribution of referral sources (this is a chart depicting the sources of referrals and the number of referrals from each source). The next step is to make a qualitative evaluation of the frequency distribution of referrals. At this point the diversity and comprehensiveness of the referral system becomes obvious. Improvements in referral sources can be planned after this qualitative evaluation has been made.

The next phase of this type of consultation concerns studying the adequacy and appropriateness of these referrals. We referred to this point above. The key question to ask is: Are the referrals in consonance with objective of the facility? If they are not, some decisions need to be made by perhaps the Board or the administrator of the facility. Part of this phase of evaluation also includes peak and valley referral load periods. In large facilities with many referral sources a frequency distribution of referrals by month of referral should be developed for each primary referral source. These distributions will provide a planning instrument to change the flow of referrals in order to increase the constancy of the referrals. To evaluate the comprehensiveness of the referral system in relation to achieving a well-balanced clientele (regularly scheduled) the consultants should develop a frequency distribution by primary disability and secondary disability. This will indicate whether the facility is in fact a multi-disability facility or a uni-disability facility.

The last phase of this type of consultation is the development of an educational program for referral sources. This public information program is developed by using the above outlined evaluations to point up the specific informational areas of each actual and potential referral source.

CASE RECORDING SYSTEMS

The case recording system is one of the most important aspects of rehabilitation facility operations and yet is also one of the most neglected. The basic purpose of all rehabilitation facilities is to facilitate the growth of clients. Facilities are goal-oriented operations. The most effective facilities develop individualized goals for each client. In order to measure growth or document growth, the facility has to have an effective case recording system. Without this case recording system the professional staff has neither documentation of the starting point in the case nor do they have an articulated end point to the process.

The case recording system which should be adopted depends upon the goals, environment, staffing pattern, and clientele of the facility; however, there is basic information required in all rehabilitation cases. A case recording system must demonstrate the basis upon which the client was accepted. This means the case folders should have all diagnostic information on the client required to understand the client's medical status and the referral problem. The case folders should have recording which states specifically the reason the client was referred. The goals of the referral source, the proposed facility activities in which the client will engage, and the goal-oriented agreement which was entered into by the referral staff and the facility staff. Consultants should be of major value in evaluating and designing case recording systems which meet these and the other needs of the specific rehabilitation facility.

NEEDS OF CLIENTS

Often a rehabilitation facility is developed by offering a very narrow spectrum of services. During the formative stages of the facility, these limited services can all be offered logically and economically. Therefore, the service program is developed around these limited services, and often the staff and Board assume they are meeting the majority of the rehabilitation needs of the clients. This attitude thwarts the normal evolutionary growth pattern of the facility. It is imperative that the needs of the clients be assessed periodically and matched against the service program of the facility. To offer less can mean that the staff does disservice to the clients of the facility.

The evaluation of client needs includes the evaluation of the prevocational sophistication of the clients through the workshop's prevocational adjustment training program. If a number of clients are in need of a prevocational adjustment training program, the consultant must ask: Does the facility have a program; if so, does the program actually raise the vocational sophistication level of the clients? Is the client actually developing a greater understanding of the relationships so necessary to become a successful worker within our culture?

If a prevocational adjustment training program is deemed necessary, a work adjustment training program is essential; however, the facility may have a work adjustment training program without having a prevocational adjustment training program. There are some key questions regarding the adequacy of the work adjustment training program. The main thrust of these questions lies in the concept that work adjustment training programs are designed to develop workmanship skills. These skills are not specific vocational skills but are skills common to all workers in competitive employment. The rehabilitation facility staff is quite often unable to make these judgments due to the closeness of their involvement in the decisions of the program services. This is an ideal role area for a technical consultant in that he brings to the facility a "fresh" point of view. He has not been involved in any of the developmental aspects of these programs nor has he participated in any of the decisions in continuing the program. Consequently he is able to evaluate decisions in terms of the service component and the relationship to the local job market.

The facility usually provides vocational evaluation services for vocational rehabilitation agencies as well as many other types of agencies. The vocational evaluation program, just as the other two programs we have discussed (the pre-vocational adjustment training program and the work adjustment training program), usually starts out on a limited basis in that it evaluates clients for rather routine low-level occupations or job families. As the facility grows and the needs of clients change, the vocational evaluation program should change also. This program (vocational evaluation) is quite susceptible to losing its relevancy to the point that it eventually evaluates clients for jobs which do not exist in significant numbers in the local job market. It is quite important that the facility staff continue to evaluate the vocational evaluation program against the criterion of value to the local job market. If clients are evaluated for jobs which are not available in their locality, generally the evaluation is a waste of time and a disservice to clients in that it builds a level of client expectation which neither the facility nor rehabilitation counselors can meet. Another fallacy in the evaluation and growth and development of vocational evaluation programs is that all too often they evaluate more for job skill training which exists in the facility than for job skills which are required in the local labor market. Consequently, if the facility has a skill training program, the staff should be cognizant of the proclivity to evaluate for the areas in which the facility can train clients. The evaluation program should be much broader than this concept. A consultant can be quite valuable in assisting facility staff in this determination both in evaluation and in skill training areas.

A program which is essential to the rehabilitation facility is the counseling program. This program has impact at all levels and in all areas of the facility. The counseling program should be initiated almost universally for rehabilitation clients. The program has many facets that should include personal and social counseling as well as vocational counseling. The personal and social counseling are needed at the beginning of the rehabilitation process, and vocational counseling spans the total process. Techniques of counseling will vary according to client needs. Both individual and group counseling may be used. A technical consultant can make a basic contribution to the facility in analyzing the counseling needs of clients and in assisting the facility in evaluating the service component through expanding or limiting counseling services as deemed appropriate.

In a new facility or a facility which is contemplating major expansion, it is wise to request a technical consultant to assist in the program expansion and program development. A consultant is prepared to assist the facility in the development of any one of five service programs—prevocational adjustment training, work adjustment training, vocational evaluation, skill training, and counseling. The consultant, then, not only is effective in analyzing the needs of clients and evaluating existing programs; he can also play a basic role in analyzing the needs of clients, anticipating the changing needs of clients, and making specific recommendations in the development of one of these programs.

STAFF DEVELOPMENT PROGRAMS

In this time of complexity, specifically in rehabilitation, we have dire need for staff development at all levels in the facility. The world of work is changing rapidly, and the rehabilitation services are changing rather rapidly. Often facility administrators recognize the need for professional upgrading; however, they neglect the paraprofessional or the subprofessional person's need for staff development. In turn, the volunteer often is neglected. The administrator should expect a consultant to work with him in the development of a comprehensive in-service training program for professional, paraprofessional and volunteer workers. A good in-service training program used to upgrade the skills of the staff should begin with three basic goals. After these goals are accomplished, then specific goals may be added to the staff development program. We will discuss in this section the general objectives of a staff development training program. The specific goals will be tailored to the needs of the staff, the level and type of clientele in the facility, and the goals and objectives of the facility.

The first goal of an in-service training program should be to change attitudes or develop attitudes regarding handicapped individuals with whom the staff is working. Attitudes toward the disabled and handicapped run the gamut from neutral to very negative. If members of the facility staff have negative views concerning the disabled, and efforts are not taken at attitude change, clients will suffer, the goals of the facility will not be achieved, and the basic mission of the facility will be subverted. Therefore, in any facility, one should carefully consider staff attitudes; if need be, work should be directed toward attitude modification.

The second goal of a staff development program is to present the goals of the facility and of rehabilitation and to teach the rehabilitation process. We have found it most interesting that a number of staff members in facilities with whom we consult have poor ideas of the goals of their facility. Their ideas of program goals are poorly articulated, rather cloudy, and quite generalized. Unless a staff member has a specific idea of the goal of that facility and the role his particular efforts play in achieving those goals, his efforts tend to be nondirected and generally ineffectual. In generalizing this to the larger field of rehabilitation, we feel that it is quite critical that rehabilitation facility personnel understand these goals of rehabilitation as well as the process of rehabilitation. If staff members are providing a service to another agency, they should understand the service program of that agency and the success criteria of that agency. Since most facilities are providing services to departments of vocational rehabilitation, the staff in the facility should understand the criteria of eligibility, the rehabilitation services, and that the only adequate end point for vocational rehabilitation is successful employment. Additionally the staff needs to know what their role is in the total rehabilitation process just as well as to know their role (specifically) with any one particular client. Without having this clear understanding, the staff member is unable to make maximum contribution.

The third area which should be included in a staff development program is the improvement of the understanding of disabilities and disabling conditions. The program which is developed with the aid of technical consultants should include material on the medical aspects of disability. This phase would offer information required to understand disabling conditions. It would include the types of medical treatment which are appropriate in the specific disabilities, types of prosthetic or orthotic appliances which are used to increase function, and expected outcome of the disability of each particular type. The second area is development of understanding of the psychological aspects of disability. One should understand the psychological impact of a disability and how an individual adjusts to that disability as well as the role that professional rehabilitation practitioners play in facilitating psychological adjustment. Thirdly, the staff development program should offer material on the functional aspects of disability. Not only should we focus on the anatomical aspects or the medical aspects of what is lost to this individual as a result of his disability, but also we should spend considerable time in discussing functional aspects. Through this approach, the staff can evaluate the residual functioning of the individual after a medical disability or psychological disability has occurred. Rehabilitation is unique in that its concern is for functional aspects of individual capability rather than the anatomical aspects. In rehabilitation, we must focus on residual functioning and how to maximize that functioning rather than on what is wrong and trying to correct what is wrong (or adjust to the disability). A consultant can play a very basic role, again, in assisting staff members with these subject areas.

ASSESSMENT OF SAFETY IN THE REHABILITATION FACILITY

Probably one of the key concerns of a rehabilitation facility administration is the safety aspect of the operation. While industries are concerned about the safety of their employees, rehabilitation facilities must pay even more attention to this aspect of operations in that the individuals involved are disabled and often adjusting to disability. These individuals are beginning a new life in the world of work, and they need to have special attention given to their work environment. A consultant should be asked specific questions about the safety of the overall operations of the facility. These questions would cover the various activity programs, the building itself, and the total physical plant. The evaluation of the safety of the facility should be in relationship to the existing facility and the current job training slots as well as to proposed job training opportunities. If the facility is expecting to make a basic change in the skill training areas or in the program of the facility, a safety consultant should be "called in" to evaluate proposed job training slots.

Another area in which a safety evaluation should be made by a consultant relates to specific disabilities. A safe work environment for a client who is mentally retarded may not be safe for someone who is blind. The consultant then will go into these various areas to evaluate the existing safety conditions and the conditions for proposed changes in program and clientele.

MODIFICATION OF JOBS AND WORK STATIONS

Another role that an outside consultant can play through a technical assistance program is that of assisting the administration and staff in the modification of jobs and work stations. Many jobs, as they are designed for industry flow systems, are inaccessible to people with certain handicaps. However, with a modification of the job (either breaking it into constituent parts or changing the order in which the job is done or by making other modifications), it becomes accessible to people with disabilities. Therefore, a consultant should be "called in" to assist in the modification of the job if a contract "hangs" in the balance or if the possibility of training and placing large numbers of clients in an industrial setting depends on modification. Related to modification jobs, is the modification of the work station in order to make it more accessible to clients with various disabilities? Whereas the first aspect of the modification of the job may be necessary to make the position more accessible, the modification of the work station allows the job to remain the same. Jigs may be constructed and provided for the disabled individual; safety gates and various types of modifications of the working environment may improve the accessibility of the disabled. A third alternative is the modification of the job and the work station to assist in making the job more accessible.

Summary

The technical assistance program has made very basic contributions to the administration and operation of rehabilitation facilities across the country; however, we find that many facility administrators who would like to use consultants are unsure of how to effectively utilize their services. This chapter has set out to discuss various ways in which a consultant can be used. There are many other roles a consultant can play. Basically, if the administration or staff is experiencing a problem or difficulties to any degree in achieving objectives of the facility, there is an indication for the need of consultation. We feel that a guiding principle should be that administrators use consultation in a positive manner to help build programs rather than just to solve problems. If a problem is anticipated, a consultant should be requested early by the administration. This allows for more effective service provision because later the problem grows to overwhelming proportions and the consultant is used to put out fires. He can be effective in the latter role as well; however, he is less effective than when used in a positive manner in planning for orderly program growth and development.

CHAPTER 11

INVOLVEMENT OF VOLUNTEERS IN REHABILITATION FACILITIES

STANLEY LEVIN *

☐ What Are the Potential Benefits of Involving Volunteers in a Rehabilitation Facility

☐ A Vital Rehabilitation Component—Someone Who Really Cares

☐ How Can An Effective Volunteer Program Be Achieved

☐ Who Are the Potential Volunteers

☐ How Much Will a Planned Volunteer Program Cost

☐ Increased Potential For Difficult Working Relationships

☐ The Challenge

THE PRESENT STATUS OF VOLUNTEERING IN REHABILITATION FACILITIES

DATA IN *The State of the Art of Volunteering in Rehabilitation Facilities* (Griggs, Levin, Obermann, 1971) indicate that 63 percent of the facilities in the United States have volunteer programs. Major strengths of these volunteer programs are briefly listed below:

1. Thousands of volunteers are involved in almost two thirds of this nation's rehabilitation facilities.
2. Volunteers are involved in a wide range of activities.

* Originally published as Why Involve Volunteers in a Rehabilitation Facility? by Goodwill Industries of America, Inc.

3. Volunteers are generally very dedicated, and they strongly believe in the programs provided by the facilities they serve.
4. About half of the volunteer programs in rehabilitation facilities have been operational for eleven years or more.
5. Appreciation for the value of volunteer participation is strongly expressed by many facility executive directors.
6. Recognition activities for volunteers are sponsored by most facilities with volunteer programs.

Despite the strengths listed above, volunteering in rehabilitation facilities has not developed to the extent of its potential. Factors responsible for the present status of volunteering in rehabilitation facilities are reviewed in the next few paragraphs.

Many executive directors and volunteers have traditionally preceived the roles of volunteers as strictly incidental to the facilities' main programs of providing rehabilitation services. Volunteers have often performed activities apart from facilities and clients, such as fund-raising projects. In those instances when volunteers have directly served clients, their participation has generally consisted of one-time special recreational or social events such as facility-sponsored picnics or holiday parties.

Positive public relations benefits have been viewed by many executive directors as the major value of volunteer participation. In fact, improved community understanding and support have frequently been considered by facility leaders to be more important than the activities and services directly performed by volunteers.

Women in the middle and upper socioeconomic strata have generally comprised the vast majority of volunteers in rehabilitation facilities. In addition to altruistic motivations for volunteering, there have been strong social considerations. Changing attitudes among, and about, women will reduce the significance of traditional social considerations in the future. Furthermore, it is very probable that future efforts to recruit volunteers for rehabilitation facilities will (and should) be extended to all segments of the population.

In traditional volunteer programs, the volunteers have participated in activities requiring skills common to most women. Typical examples of these activities are: organizing fund-raising events, such as home tours, antique sales, card parties, and teas; preparing food for special occasions; planning games and entertainment for clients' social and recreational events. Frequently, volunteers have been assigned jobs that require minimal skills, such as stuffing, stamping, and sorting direct mail pieces; delivering or picking up materials and equipment; routine telephoning. These jobs are not to be considered unimportant, and must be continued as long as they meet needs vital to the functioning of rehabilitation facilities. However, volunteer involvement in activities like those just described barely taps the potential benefits available to facilities and clients through PLANNED VOLUNTEER PROGRAMS.

If volunteering in rehabilitation facilities is to progress beyond present levels of productivity, and if the quality of volunteering is to improve, Executive Directors and other leaders of facilities must take a fresh look at the potentials of volunteer participation in relation to their facilities' purposes. Also, they must reevaluate operational practices presently performed in relation to key components of their volunteer programs, such as identifying and outlining volunteer jobs, recruiting, interviewing, training and supervising.

WHAT ARE THE POTENTIAL BENEFITS OF INVOLVING VOLUNTEERS IN A REHABILITATION FACILITY?

Volunteer involvement in a rehabilitation facility can substantially help achieve the goal of the rehabilitation process. The following benefits can be realized within any particular facility which institutes a PLANNED VOLUNTEER PROGRAM:

1. Increased services to handicapped and disadvantaged clients.
2. Bridging clients from the facility to the community.
3. A vital rehabilitation component—someone who really cares.
4. Community understanding and cooperation.
5. Social action.
6. Fund raising.

7. Administrative and clerical assistance.
8. Technical assistance and professional consultation.
9. Bringing people together.

Increased Services to Handicapped and Disadvantaged Clients

Through the involvement of carefully trained and constructively supervised volunteers in the delivery of rehabilitation services, more time can be devoted to clients by paid professional and technical staff members. An expanded variety of services can be made available to clients and other handicapped persons. Facility clients can experience more individualized rehabilitation services.

MORE TIME FOR CLIENTS. Volunteers can be of great assistance to paid personnel of a facility by performing a number of activities, such as filling out reports, client scheduling, phone calls, correspondence, and meeting arrangements. Although important, these activities need not require the personal attention of skilled staff members. Paid facility personnel, relieved of certain time-consuming tasks, can devote a greater percentage of their energy and talents to providing clients with professional services, such as counseling, instruction, testing, and therapeutic treatment.

Of equal importance and consequence in providing increased professional time for individual clients, is the practice of involving volunteers who are qualified practitioners in areas of rehabilitation programming. Far too often, volunteers are erroneously considered untrained and lacking in professional credentials or technical skills. There are many people in this country with academic degrees in psychology, nursing, social work, speech therapy, education, and other fields, who are retired, temporarily inactive, or working only part-time. These capable persons should be recruited to volunteer four hours per week (or more) in programs in which they can apply their specialized knowledge and experience. Not only do most qualified persons in these circumstances prefer to more fully utilize their skills and contribute to society, but many professionally inactive individuals are interested in maintaining high levels of proficiency in their specialties.

Through the effective involvement of either type of volunteer described above, it will be possible for more professional time to be devoted to a given number of clients, or for more clients to receive professional services, or both.

EXPANDED VARIETY OF SERVICES FOR CLIENTS. Volunteers can expand the range of services a facility can provide, and thereby enrich the total rehabilitation program. Through productive recruitment efforts, persons with special talents can become involved on a voluntary basis and institute activities that would otherwise be unavailable. Volunteers often bring unusual skills and devote many hours of service that enrich the total facility program through such projects as personal grooming, music and art, one-to-one educational assistance, an on-the-premises library, social and recreational events, and consumer education. Many of these additional services are of special value to clients as they endeavor to become more integrated into their communities.

MORE INDIVIDUALIZED PROGRAMS FOR CLIENTS. One very important result of additional professional time, and an expanded variety of services being available, is the increased opportunity to design rehabilitation programs which more precisely meet particular needs of individual clients of the facility. Strengthening the degree to which rehabilitation programs are personalized should improve the effectiveness of the entire rehabilitation process.

Bridging Clients From the Facility to the Community

Many rehabilitation authorities and facility leaders recognize the urgent need to transfer substantial components of rehabilitation programming from facility settings to community settings. Rehabilitation services have not moved more extensively in this direction because of many difficult factors. It is one process to counsel and assist a client within the jurisdiction of a facility, and to hypothetically discuss life and realities within the larger community. Another approach must necessarily be applied if the client actually is to be introduced to the environment of the larger community, and is to be required to learn through direct exposure and experience. The latter approach requires rehabilitation leaders and personnel to work closely with people within the larger community in the arranging of positive opportunities for handicapped persons to become accustomed to "new" social or employment situations.

One of the best ways to help clients bridge the chasms between the security of their facilities and the uncertainties of mainstream society is through volunteer participation. As rehabilitation facilities work more closely with the larger community, the citizenry can begin to better understand how to help handicapped and disadvantaged persons become assimilated into existing social and economic structures. Volunteers who work directly with facilities can lead the way.

For example, volunteers could take groups of clients to a nearby public library, acquaint them with the range of library services, assist them with securing library cards, and help them learn how to locate books of special interest. Public transportation could be used to travel from the facility to the library, thereby providing the clients with experience in use of public transit systems. Certain clients might be encouraged to enroll in special classes which are often sponsored by municipal libraries or public school systems. Through such activities, clients can become acquainted with other members of the community and have "joining" or social experiences of special value. Another example could involve a college music sorority inviting facility clients with special talent or fondness for music to participate in particular programs or events—sometimes as spectators, and other times as performers.

This kind of client involvement within the larger community, made possible through volunteers, should help members of the general public gain greater understanding of the capabilities and needs of facility clients. Through increased public understanding, the housing, transportation, accessibility, placement, and social needs of all handicapped and disadvantaged persons will likely be more fully recognized and more completely met. In addition, this form of interaction with the community can help clients apply what they have learned at the facility to practical daily living.

A VITAL REHABILITATION COMPONENT—SOMEONE WHO REALLY CARES

People going through the rehabilitation process need to have their feelings of personal worth strengthened. They must feel that their personal thoughts, talents, and knowledge are appreciated by other people. These feelings foster the spirit of hopefulness that is a powerful force without which rehabilitation cannot occur within an individual.

An essential, and often overlooked, element in the total rehabilitation process is the special kind of caring that generates and reinforces feelings of hope. This kind of caring cannot be purchased at any price because its essence is imbedded in its being given freely. It can only be extended by people who voluntarily give it, whether they are paid staff or volunteers.

Clients have expressed receiving great encouragement from volunteers who, they know, are not being paid to care about them. Kindness, understanding, and honest friendship willingly given to clients by volunteers can be as important as the most capably provided professional service. Thus, their special kind of caring can be one of the greatest benefits infused into the rehabilitation process by volunteers working directly with clients.

Community Understanding and Cooperation

Volunteers maintain important relationships within neighborhoods and communities. Their connections with churches, service clubs, and other associations can be of great value in terms of increasing public awareness about the facilities in which they participate. As they circulate informally among neighbors and friends, and attend organized events, volunteers can effectively disseminate information about rehabilitation facilities and handicapped persons. They can improve the public's image of facilities through conversations or discussions in which they explain operational procedures, cite disabilities served, correct misconceptions or false reports, and project success stories. Equally effective are formal presentations by volunteers to groups such as civic clubs or professional associations. A positive public image that in enhanced through volunteer participation has provided benefits in the form of monetary contributions and increased levels of morale among paid staff and clients served.

Volunteers who acquire knowledge about different agencies, or who become aware of similar programs within their communities, have been successful in fostering interorganizational communication and helping bring about interagency cooperation. Among the benefits that can result from volunteer-assisted coordination of efforts, is the opportunity for rehabilitation facilities to arrange more complete service programs than would generally be possible if each facility duplicated similar services. Because community leaders react favorably to cooperative endeavors that simultaneously reduce duplication and achieve more comprehensive service, the rehabilitation of handicapped and disadvantaged persons receives more positive response and increased status when there is widespread awareness of interagency coordination.

Social Action

Handicapped and disadvantaged persons need advocates who are willing to speak out on matters which significantly affect their ability to support themselves; to live independently; to enjoy cultural, educational, and social opportunities. Volunteers who have salient facts and strong convictions can be very instrumental in bringing about constructive societal changes.

Volunteers have demonstrated their capabilities to increase society's awareness of many situations of serious consequence to the national health and welfare. Voluntary social action is not limited to the dissemination of information, nor to the federal government scene. Forms of voluntary action include supporting or opposing legislation, and influencing formulation or revision of policies—at the local, state, and national levels.

Fund Raising

Fund-raising efforts of volunteers are very closely related to the degree of public understanding present within the community. Successful community fund raising generally results from widespread agreement with the facility's purpose, and public belief in competent facility operation. Certainly, the raising of money is much easier if a facility has positive public and community relations.

Communitywide drives may seek funds for capital and/or operational needs of a facility. Specific projects might be organized to raise money for special needs of individual clients. Groups of volunteers, such as auxiliaries or service organizations, have exhibited proficiency in conducting profitable fund-raising activities.

Administrative and Clerical Assistance

Volunteers, especially those with the appropriate skills and experience, can perform all types of administrative and clerical assignments. Compiling statistical reports, maintaining records, procuring contract work, helping with mailings and filing, and preparing annual reports are a few of the many ways in which volunteers can assist the general operations of a rehabilitation facility.

TECHNICAL ASSISTANCE AND PROFESSIONAL CONSULTATION

All communities include people who have technical knowledge and skills, or professional capabilities and expertise, that can be of immeasurable value to rehabilitation facilities and their clients. For example, writers, artists, marketing experts, personnel specialists, and interior decorators might assist with specific projects of importance to facility operation. Or, architects, accountants, engineers, medical specialists, and university faculty members might become involved in particular activities related to general facility functions or individual client needs. If called upon, most technical and professional persons are usually willing to provide reasonable amounts of advice, consultation, or assistance to a recognized rehabilitation facility serving handicapped and disadvantaged persons.

Bringing People Together

In addition to the facility and its clients, volunteer service in a rehabilitation facility benefits the volunteers. Indeed, for many volunteers, the "need to help others" and the "need to be needed" are met through the personal satisfaction and fulfillment they receive when they serve humanity in a worthwhile, meaningful way. In this repect, rehabilitation facilities offer settings in which people can dramatically and significantly help each other.

Through volunteer service, people are able to gain greater insight into the problems and lives of other human beings. As a result of this insight, they often take actions that help correct inequities existing within society. As a result of volunteer participation, many people gain courage, strength, humility, and appreciation for their personal circumstances. Through volunteer involvement, people can develop better perspectives of their own lives and values. In these respects, rehabilitation facilities serve volunteers too.

Thus, volunteering adds a powerful dimension to the programs of rehabilitation facilities. By bringing together clients of facilities and "nonhandicapped" people of the community, volunteering extends benefits beyond the clients, beyond the facility, even beyond the participating volunteers. This bringing people together benefits society by facilitating social renewal. The more people are brought together, the more they realize how similar and mutually interdependent all lives are, regardless of certain personal circumstances. As this realization deepens, there is increased potential for more complete rehabilitation of handicapped and disadvantaged persons. As this realization widens, there is greater potential for societal rehabilitation and progress toward humanity's highest goals.

HOW CAN AN EFFECTIVE VOLUNTEER PROGRAM BE ACHIEVED?

In a series of handbooks recently published by Goodwill Industries of America, the essential components of a

PLANNED VOLUNTEER PROGRAM are outlined and described in considerable detail. (See list of handbook titles at end of this chapter.) Implementing these components should produce an effective volunteer program that can help a rehabilitation facility accomplish the benefits previously mentioned. Concisely summarized, a PLANNED VOLUNTEER PROGRAM features the following:

1. Thorough organization.
2. Competent administration.
3. Positive attitudes.
4. Creativity.

Thorough Organization

Effective volunteer programs do not just happen. They require planning and systematic follow-up. General organizational principles practiced in relation to other program components of a rehabilitation facility must also be applied to the development of a volunteer program.

A PLANNED VOLUNTEER PROGRAM must incorporate certain components and procedures to attain operational efficiency and high-quality results:

1. Volunteer Job Descriptions.
2. Recruitment.
3. Interviewing.
4. Placement.
5. Preparation (Orientation and Training programs).
6. Supervision.
7. Evaluation.
8. Recognition.

Competent Administration

Similar to any department within a facility, a volunteer program requires capable administrative leadership. A qualified person should be appointed to the position of Director of Volunteer Services. Whether this person works full-time or part-time, he should have department head status, and be clearly perceived as an extension of the Executive Director. Volunteers must receive supervision in the same manner as paid staff members. When volunteers work with rehabilitation programs and directly relate to clients, constructive supervision becomes extremely important.

Positive Attitudes

Leaders of rehabilitation facilities must strongly believe in the values and advantages of volunteer participation. Particular, Executive Directors need to frequently express firm convictions about the benefits which can result from volunteer efforts. They must be able to see beyond the current stage of volunteering, and be able to envision the great potential resources that volunteer involvement can contribute to the rehabilitation of handicapped and disadvantaged persons.

Also of considerable importance is the existence of positive attitudes toward the volunteer program among a facility's governing body, its paid staff members, and its clients. It is necessary that they all understand the scope, purposes, and operations of the facility's volunteer program.

Creativity

It is unlikely that a PLANNED VOLUNTEER PROGRAM will be inaugurated or maintained without the infusion and encouragement of creative ideas. What kinds of creativity will be needed? Creative leadership which will increase understanding of, and enthusiasm for, volunteer participation among the facility's paid staff. Imaginative thinking about volunteer jobs and assignments. Innovative techniques for recruiting volunteers from all segments of society in sufficient quantity, and with appropriate qualifications, to meet the needs of the facility and its clients. Creative approaches for bringing volunteers, clients, and paid staff members together in more meaningful relationships.

Idealism and creativity should not be inhibited in a volunteer program. Ideas that might have originally seemed unrealistic may turn out to be highly practical and worthwhile.

WHO ARE THE POTENTIAL VOLUNTEERS?

Everyone. But not everyone for every job. Volunteers must be carefully interviewed, selected, and placed in appropriate assignments.

Certain individuals in a given community will have to be personally recruited and encouraged to contribute their special knowledge or skills. Constituting a large pool of untapped volunteer manpower are young people, minority group members, business and professional persons, retired individuals, members of organized labor and handicapped and disadvantaged persons. In addition, Community Organizations can be approached and invited to assume particular responsibilities within a rehabilitation facility. Such organizations include civic and service clubs, professional associations, religious groups, sororities and fraternal or veterans organizations, hobby clubs, and groups with special recreational or social interests. Of course, auxiliaries and other types of Facility Organizations, which exist exclusively to provide volunteer service to particular facilities, have long been major sources of volunteers.

Many people, who heretofore have not been extensively involved in volunteer programs, can be of considerable value to rehabilitation facilities. For example, unique services can be provided by handicapped volunteers, such as providing information and guidance regarding prosthetics, helping with driver training instruction, and serving as spokesmen for a facility and its clients throughout the community. A group of handicapped persons could advise facility leaders on program relevancy and program effectiveness.

HOW MUCH WILL A PLANNED VOLUNTEER PROGRAM COST?

A very pervasive misconception is that volunteer programs do not, and should not, cost money. When many people hear the word, "volunteer," they immediately think about efforts and activities that do not involve the expenditure of funds; that are "free" of costs. They assume that volunteers, through some mystical process, can participate in the operation and program of a rehabilitation facility without the involvement of paid staff in training and supervising, without any allocation for supplies and materials, and without providing volunteers with out-of-pocket expenses. Of course, these assumptions are erroneous and unrealistic.

It is correct that a major benefit of volunteer participation is the provision of increased services and more individualized attention for clients than would otherwise be available within most facilities. It is also factual that volunteers frequently raise substantial funds for rehabilitation facilities. However, it is invalid to conclude that these benefits result from activities that do not require the expenditure of monies or the allocation of other resources. Facility leaders must recognize the necessity, and be willing, to invest money and other resources in order to obtain the advantages of volunteer participation.

It is important to note that many Executive Directors believe the benefits to facilities and clients, from a well-planned and capably administered volunteer program, can more than compensate for the costs involved. In some facilities, volunteers raise more money than the combined total of direct and indirect volunteer program costs. A number of facility leaders have calculated that the dollar value of voluntarily contributed services far exceeds the total costs of operating their volunteer programs. Many Executive Directors believe the favorable public relations and increased community goodwill more than justify the costs of maintaining volunteer programs.

Costs of any particular volunteer program will depend on the nature of the rehabilitation facility and the scope of its service program. However, most PLANNED VOLUNTEER PROGRAMS, regardless of size or nature, will involve certain *direct* and *indirect* costs:

Direct Costs of Planned Volunteer Programs:

1. Office supplies and equipment.
2. Salary and fringe benefits for a Director of Volunteer Services. (In certain situations, this position may be filled by a volunteer.)
3. General and specific materials related to volunteer Orientation and Training programs, recruitment efforts, recognition activities, etc.
4. Reimbursement of personal expenses incurred by volunteers in conjunction with their participation, such as parking, mileage, meals, registration fees, etc.
5. Insurance coverage for volunteers.
6. Expenses related to Assigned activities, such as tickets to sports or cultural events, special transportation costs, etc.

Indirect Costs of Planned Volunteer Programs:

1. Time of the Executive Director and Paid staff members required for planning, interviewing, training, supervising, and other operational activities.
2. Office space, heat, lights, and use of equipment.
3. Secretarial assistance. (Volunteers may provide this assistance.)

WHAT DIFFICULTIES OR PROBLEMS MIGHT BE INVOLVED IN A PLANNED VOLUNTEER PROGRAM?

Difficulties are experienced in any endeavor important to the improvement of human welfare. A PLANNED VOLUNTEER PROGRAM is no exception.

Increased Complexity of a Facility Program

From a managerial standpoint, the involvement of volunteers to assist with existing operations and to add new services will increase administrative responsibilities. There will be more people to supervise and coordinate. Growth in the rehabilitation program will require additional space and materials. Scheduling client activities will become increasingly complicated as efforts are made to take advantage of recreational and cultural events that occur throughout the community during or after normal facility operating hours. As a rehabilitation program expands and becomes more multifaceted, the entire operation of a rehabilitation facility becomes more complex. More frequent communication, and increased emphasis on coordination and cooperation, can help reduce unproductive by-products of an increasingly complex facility program.

Liability for Actions of Volunteers

The extent to which facilities can be held liable for the actions of volunteers should receive prompt and serious consideration. Additional or special types of insurance coverage may be necessary to adequately protect a facility and its volunteers. While national attention is increasingly being focused on this subject, matters of liability and insurance vary according to state laws. Therefore, specialized legal and insurance consultation should be sought in order to comply with local requirements.

Additional Operating Costs

Direct costs of a PLANNED VOLUNTEER PROGRAM were outlined in the previous section of this chapter. Finding additional money, regardless of how it will be expended, is generally a problem for most rehabilitation facilities. Direct costs of the volunteer program should be built into the operating budget of the facility. This practice evidences acceptance of the principle that the volunteer program is an integral part of the facility's total operation.

Usual sources of funds should not be overlooked as means of financing part, or all, of a PLANNED VOLUNTEER PROGRAM. In addition, some facilities may have special sources of funding available, depending on local circumstances.

Civic and service organizations might underwrite all, or certain, of the costs of a volunteer program. In some communities, particular organizations or local foundations will provide funds to help inaugurate new services on the basis of gradually reducing support. This often means an organization or foundation will totally finance a new service, project, or program for the first year; meet 50 percent of the costs during the second year; and provide 25 percent of the budget for the third year. Usually it is agreed that the service or program will be financed —after the third year—on the same basis as other vital community services. In some instances, certain governmental agencies are able to provide funds, through grants or purchase of service contracts, that can help meet facility operating costs.

INCREASED POTENTIAL FOR DIFFICULT WORKING RELATIONSHIPS

The possibility that tension and strained working relationships may develop between volunteers and paid staff members is another difficulty that must be realistically considered. Some paid staff members may feel their job security is threatened by the participation of nonpaid persons. When a facility involves volunteers from all segments of the population, differing value orientations and life styles can cause conflict and troublesome interaction.

The problem of difficult working relationships is rooted in negative attitudes harbored by both paid staff and volunteers. A number of measures can minimize, if not prevent, the development of this problem. Basic to positive working relationships is mutual understanding of each other's roles, and mutual respect for each other's contributions to the facility's program. The purpose and operation of the volunteer program should be carefully explained to all paid staff, with assurances that volunteers augment the activities of paid staff but under no circumstances supplant them. Application of the principles and procedures basic to a PLANNED VOLUNTEER PROGRAM will increase the probabilities for pleasant and productive working relationships flourishing among paid staff and volunteers.

Additional Potentially Disruptive Situations

It is important that consideration also be given to other realities of a volunteer program operation that sometimes become minor (or major) problems for leaders of rehabilitation facilities.

Volunteers often bring an "outside" perspective into the facilities they serve. Their intent to improve the programs with which they identify may prompt them to offer proposals and recommendations for changes in the volunteer program or in the facilities' operational procedures and policies. Sometimes volunteers can become overly energetic or very zealous in their questioning of policies and pursuit of change. This type of activity, regardless of intent, can be upsetting to paid staff and clients, and can be considered disruptive to the facilities' operations.

On the other hand, many executive directors of facilities that involve volunteers consider the introduction of new ideas and suggestions to be a positive stimulant that prevents stagnation and reduces complaceny. Questioning and the offering of recommendations are encouraged through joint participative activities and organized channels. In these settings, facility leaders value enthusiastic and imaginative volunteers for the increased and improved programs they generate. Volunteers are often compared to a fresh breeze, and are recognized as a source of creative energy that helps facilities maintain dynamic growth and progress.

Some volunteers have difficulty fitting into the organizational pattern of the facility; they fail to comply with facility policies and regulations or to participate in training programs; and some disregard staff guidance and instructions. Certain volunteers are unreliable about reporting for assignments at specified places or times, while other volunteers are not consistent in the quality of their work or the completion of tasks on schedule.

Fortunately, only a small proportion of volunteers reflect the characteristics described above. Most of those who may exhibit one or more such traits early in their volunteer careers usually respond to leadership actions that help them realize the consequences of their behavior, and they begin to act more constructively. This emphasizes the necessity for strong leaders who perceive, and help volunteers to understand, that volunteers must function as unpaid employees of the facility.

Preventing, or minimizing, potentially disruptive volunteer behavior can be accomplished through soundly organized and capably conducted Orientation and Training programs. Poorly instructed volunteers can be expected to generate the same kind of problems as poorly instructed paid staff members. Recognition of this reality reinforces the advantages of involving paid staff and volunteers, together, in certain activities designed to prepare personnel for participation in the facility program. A Volunteer Manual and other informational materials can be distributed to help each volunteer more fully understand facility policies and volunteer program procedures. Application of constructive supervision by both key paid staff members and volunteer leaders will encourage productive performance. Frequent expressions of appreciation, and other appropriate types of informal or formal recognition, promote positive attitudes and effectively motivate individuals to improve their efforts.

Difficulties and problems are not unique to the organization and operation of volunteer programs. Most of the situations identified in the last several paragraphs occur within all agencies, facilities, institutions, and organizations regardless of size or setting. It is possible to prevent many problems from happening; it is feasible to reduce or reverse the impact of most difficult and unproductive circumstances. Principal tools for prevention or reduction of undesirable situations are: careful planning, skillful organization, competent administration, adequate preparation, constructive supervision, and flexible implementation.

THE CHALLENGE

One of the great challenges confronting contemporary leaders concerns providing all individuals with opportunities to participate in the events and activities of our society. Rehabilitation facilities represent one of the principal vehicles for enabling people to realize their highest potentials for living and participating in mainstream social and economic structures. Through the rehabilitation process, handicapped and disadvantaged persons are helped to attain new levels of dignity and stronger feelings of self-worth and purpose. This process recognizes the need people have for association with other people, and the desire of people to help others. In other words, rehabilitation applies the fundamental principle of mutual helpfulness. At the heart of this principle is volunteerism.

Volunteerism is a missing component in many rehabilitation facilities, and is not highly developed in the majority of facilities. By increasing the involvement of volunteers in their facilities, and by improving the quality of their volunteer programs, leaders of rehabilitation facilities have an unusual opportunity to expand the entire scope and effectiveness of the rehabilitation process. In addition, through PLANNED VOLUNTEER PROGRAMS, leaders of rehabilitation facilities are in an extraordinary position to increase the opportunities for, and the abilities of, more people to participate meaningfully in our society.

REFERENCES

The titles listed below are available through Goodwill Industries of America, Inc., National Auxiliary to Goodwill Industries, 9200 Wisconsin Avenue, Washington, D. C. 20014. These handbooks were prepared as part of Research and Demonstration Grant #12-P-55087/3-03, Rehabilitation Services Administration, Social and Rehabilitation Service, U. S. Department of Health, Education and Welfare. The project was sponsored by Goodwill Industries of America, Inc., and the National Auxiliary to Goodwill Industries.

1. WHY INVOLVE VOLUNTEERS
in a Rehabilitation Facility
2. HOW TO ORGANIZE A VOLUNTEER PROGRAM
in a Rehabilitation Facility
3. HOW VOLUNTEERS CAN HELP
in a Rehabilitation Facility
4. HOW TO ADMINISTER A VOLUNTEER PROGRAM
in a Rehabilitation Facility
5. HOW TO RECRUIT VOLUNTEERS
in a Rehabilitation Facility
6. HOW TO INTERVIEW AND PLACE VOLUNTEERS
in a Rehabilitation Facility
7. HOW TO PREPARE VOLUNTEERS TO HELP
in a Rehabilitation Facility
8. HOW TO SUPERVISE AND EVALUATE VOLUNTEERS
in a Rehabilitation Facility
9. HOW TO MOTIVATE VOLUNTEERS
in a Rehabilitation Facility
10. HOW TO INCORPORATE GROUP VOLUNTEERING
in a Rehabilitation Facility
11. HOW TO ASSURE RESPONSIBLE VOLUNTEERING
in a Rehabilitation Facility
12. CATALOG OF RESOURCES
Volunteers in Rehabilitation Facilities

OTHER RESOURCE MATERIAL

Hardy, Richard E. and Cull, John G.: APPLIED VOLUNTEERISM IN COMMUNITY DEVELOPMENT, Charles C Thomas, Publisher, 1974.

Cull, John G. and Hardy, Richard E.: VOLUNTEERISM: AN EMERGING PROFESSION, Charles C Thomas, Publisher, 1973.

REFERENCES

Griggs, Robert J., Levin, Stanley, and Obermann, C. Esco: *The State of the Art of Volunteering in Rehabilitation Facilities.* Washington, D. C.: Goodwill Industries of America, Inc. and National Auxiliary to Goodwill Industries, 1971, p. 8.

CHAPTER 12

CONSIDERATIONS IN THE DEVELOP-MENT OF A PLACEMENT PROGRAM IN REHABILITATION FACILITIES

RICHARD E. HARDY AND JOHN G. CULL

☐ A Science of Vocational Behavior

☐ Client-Centered Placement

☐ Developing an Employment Program

☐ Five Questions Counselors Must Be Able to Answer

☐ Some Guidelines and Tools in Locating Employment Opportunities

☐ Professional Placement

☐ Getting the Client Ready for Employment

☐ Relating Psychological Data to Job Analysis Information in Vocational Placement

O NE OF THE MOST SUBSTANTIAL contributions a rehabilitation facility can make which affects the client's overall mental and physical adjustment is the preparation of the client for placement on a job that is well-suited to his abilities and interests. Vocational placement is underrated by many rehabilitationists and others who do not understand the full effects of its outcome. Helping the client find employment is often relegated to scanning newspaper want ads in search of opportunities or responding to a call from an employer who happens to have an available job. Certainly occupational opportunities can be located through these means. However, the matching of the individual and the job is a complicated process which requires careful study and evaluation through inter-relating all casework data on the individual with all information that can be secured relating to job requirements and job setting.

A SCIENCE OF VOCATIONAL BEHAVIOR

Loftquist and Davis (1969) discussed a "science of vocational behavior" which they see as essentially vocational psychology. Whether one agrees or not that the "science of vocational behavior" is actually vocational psychology, the necessity for the full development of vocational behavior study as a science cannot be overstressed. The substantial growth during recent years of interest in the Vocational Evaluation and Work Adjustment Division of the National Rehabilitation Association and the subsequent publication of the Vocational Evaluation and Work Adjustment Bulletin have done a great deal to stimulate thinking and research on vocational behavior and practical problems of the individual and groups in the world of work. Certainly, in the future, vocational adjustment studies and work evaluation will take an even more prominent place in the rehabilitation counselor's work and in rehabilitation counselor education within the university settings.

Above all, rehabilitation facility personnel must be able to understand the "work personality" of clients in the facility. The "work personality profile" consists of such factors as vocational and avocational interests, abilities, needs, work habits, psychological maturity and interaction with on-the-job factors including job hierarchies, communication and health factors.

One of the prime concerns in the development of the rehabilitation facility should be for the vocational objective of the clientele. This requires the development of expertise in placement. The staff should become familiar with available research on work adjustment and should be familiar with the studies done in vocational rehabilitation at the University of Minnesota since 1957. These studies offer a great deal of useful information regarding work adjustment and work placement or vocational placement.

CLIENT-CENTERED PLACEMENT

Rehabilitationists have heard much about "client-centered counseling" over the years. Because placement is an important part of the rehabilitation process, counselors should think of "client-centered placement." Job placement is a major client service which has helped rehabilitation agencies in getting substantial amounts of federal and state funds for program operations. The goal of work is one of the unique characteristics of rehabilitation. The placement of individuals on jobs through which they can find methods to maintain themselves is the concept which has allowed rehabilitation counseling to gain in stature as a social service profession with a substantial contribution to make to the individual and to society. In fact, most laymen would probably say that the location of appropriate jobs for clients is the main function of the rehabilitation staff and facilities. It is interesting that rehabilitation staff downplay the importance of placement in their jobs when they describe their activities to their friends and colleagues. Counselors might reflect more seriously upon their placement responsibilities if clients were thought of as consumers of their services and were given an opportunity to actually evaluate the jobs which they have obtained with the help of the counselor.

In fact, the use of the phrase "PLACE in employment" is one which misleads the rehabilitation staff trainee and others concerning the method which should be used. The client and counselor must work together in order for the client to reach a decision concerning the type of job he wishes to have. After this decision is made and the rehabilitation staff and facility helps the client secure information about various jobs that exist in the geographical area where he wants to be employed, the client himself should take some initiative whenever possible to get employment with the assistance of the counselor. Once a feasible job is located, the client should be given the opportunity to evaluate it as the source of his future livelihood.

Quite often, when considering placement, the counselor is confronted with the dilemma of determining to whom he owes basic loyalty—the client or the employer—that is, should he be protective of the client when dealing with an employer or protective of the employer. How much of the client's problems and disability should the counselor relate to the employer? Should he obscure the client's disability in discussions with the employer?

If the professional relationship was bilateral and concerned only the client and counselor the answer to the dilemma would be immediately obvious; however, the relationship is trilateral.

Client

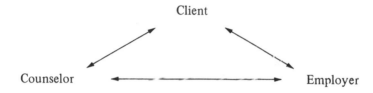

Counselor   Employer

As such, the counselor owes equal professional responsibility to both the client and prospective employer. Therefore, the counselor should communicate with the employer in a basic, forthright manner. The counselor is professionally obligated to be honest in his dealings with the employer.

If the counselor fails to be completely honest and forthright with the employer, he not only jeopardizes his professional relationship with this employer thereby obviating any possibility of placing clients in this area in the future, but he also takes a great chance of jeopardizing the client-employer relationship later when the employer becomes more aware of the client's attributes which the counselor chose to hide or misrepresent. Consequently, I feel rather strongly that the counselor should discuss with the client what he is planning to relate to the employer. If the client refuses to allow the counselor to discuss his assets, liabilities and disability with the employer, the counselor should modify his role in the placement process.

His role should be one of providing placement information to the client, but he should not enter actively into the placement process with the client.

There are two limits to this interchange between the counselor and employer relative to the client:

1. The counselor and employer should discuss thoroughly those aspects and only those aspects of the client's background which have a direct relation with the job.
2. The counselor should communicate with the employer on a level at which both are comfortable in the exchange of information.

Quite often a counselor approaches a prospective employer regarding a specific client and as the conversation progresses the counselor finds himself relating information which, while highly pertinent in the rehabilitation process, has little to do with the client as an employee. In each instance in which the counselor makes an employer contact for placement purposes, the counselor should have summarized previously all material in the case folder which is directly related to the client's proficiency in a particular position—both his assets and liabilities. After reviewing this summary the counselor should refrain from relating any other information he may have derived from counseling sessions, training evaluations or diagnostic work-ups. A mark of professionalism is the ability to communicate the essential factors relating to the client and still respect the client's fundamental right to confidentiality of case material.

The second limitation to communication between the counselor and employer requires the counselor to assess the sophistication of the employer and communicate with him on that level. As a general rule the counselor should avoid using terminology which, though descriptive, is highly laden with emotional connotations. The most effective approach the counselor can take in discussing the client's assets and liabilities is to describe behavior rather than categorizing it with diagnostic labels. For example, this person experienced learning difficulties in the academic areas rather early and is slow in learning new procedures. He is ineffective in dealing with abstract concepts and carrying out complex, oral instructions and should not be placed in a situation requiring independent judgments in changing conditions; however, he is very adept in performing concrete tasks and is capable of making routine, repetitive judgments. This description means more to the employer than the term "mental retardate."

DEVELOPING AN EMPLOYMENT PROGRAM

Counselors who are involved with placement should be familiar with information offered in the publication, *Workers Worth Their Hire* (American Mutual Insurance Alliance), which is available through the President's Committee on Employment of the Physically Handicapped. Myths concerning employment of the handicapped are disspelled by information given in this publication. Counselors will find that discussions of the excellent record of handicapped persons in such areas as safety, absenteeism, production and motivation to work are of considerable help to them in their discussions with employers, union leaders and work supervisors. The counselor should be certain that he not only talks about these factors with top agency employment officials but also that he manages, at the appropriate time, to mention these subjects to supervisors within the work area. The degree of acceptance which supervisors give to handicapped clients is often influential in not only helping them "get off to a good start" but also in maintaining their work at a level commensurate with the supervisor's expectations.

Some rehabilitation staff and facilities have felt that the counselor should not have a specific client in mind when talking with an employer, but that he should sell the concept of hiring the handicapped to the employer and later get into the work setting in order to locate the types of jobs which would be available to handicapped individuals. This concept can be extremely useful and can help open many doors to handicapped employees; however, after convincing the employer of the value of hiring handicapped persons, the counselor often will be asked to refer a prospective employee immediately if a particular opening exists in the work setting. If a counselor is unable to meet this request, his public relations and sales program can be substantially damaged in terms of future placements with the employer.

Each rehabilitation staff and facility should constantly evaluate his efforts in placement to make certain that he is moving clients toward jobs in line with their overall adjustment and ability. One of the key sources of learning about job opportunities for any client is often the client's past experiences and previous job responsibilities. In many cases, clients will wish to return to the type of employment held prior to the onset of the employment handicap. In fact, many former employers will feel a responsibility for injured employees and wish again to offer them employment after they have received rehabilitation services. The client will offer many insights about himself to the counselor who then has the responsibility to match abilities, needs and interests of the client with requirements and offerings of the job. One of the primary sources, then, of information about types of employment for the client is the client himself. This information can be gained by a study of his background and from interest inventories and interviews with him and his family.

The counselor will also wish to use the services of the state employment agency which maintains local offices throughout the United States. Many prospective employers inform the employment service of job openings. This agency also offers counseling, placement and evaluation services for handicapped job applicants. The Vocational Rehabilitation Act, Public Law 89-565 stipulates that the vocational rehabilitation state plan shall "provide for entering into cooperative agreements with the system of public employment offices in the state and the maximum utilization of the job placement and employment counseling services and other services and facilities of such offices."

FIVE QUESTIONS COUNSELORS MUST BE ABLE TO ANSWER

Of course, many different problem areas can arise when the counselor is discussing hiring handicapped workers with an employer. Questions range from, How will the person get to the place of employment? to What will he do in case of fire? Incidentally, these two questions usually can be answered with the same responses which any employee would give—in the first case, "By bus or car" and in the second, "Get the hell out like everyone else."

The first basic question which usually arises is that of increased insurance rates if handicapped workers are employed. This is most often an honest employer reaction to the question concerning employment of handicapped workers. Insurance rates would rise if individuals were employed in an agency which tended to have more accidents; however, handicapped workers have been proven to be as safe in the performance of their duties as other workers. In fact, some handicapped persons such as the blind have actually shown better records of safety than nonhandicapped workers. American Mutual Insurance Alliance has published materials relevant to the fact that handicapped workers are as safe or safer than nonhandicapped workers. The counselor should have this information readily available and indicate to the prospective employer that indeed workmen's compensation insurance rates are determined, in part, according to the relative hazards of the work done by the industry in question. Yearly rates also are determined according to the industry's record of accidents and insurance claims. These are good reasons for hiring handicapped workers. If an employer persists in believing that his insurance rates will increase, the counselor should ask him to contact his insurance agent or read again his insurance contract.

A second question which often arises is this: Why should I hire a handicapped individual when I can employ "normal" persons whom I can count on for employment without difficulty? The counselor will have to answer this question according to his own philosophy and training. Some helpful responses might include the following:

1. Ask why he should not employ individuals whose employment records have been proven and who are well known and highly recommended by rehabilitation and employment specialists.
2. Describe the medical, social and psychiatric evaluations completed on all clients (not being specific or violating confidentiality). In

other words, why not hire an individual who comes to the employer, in a sense, "certified" as ready for employment?

3. Remind him that by doing so he is actually supporting what he, as a taxpayer, has already invested some money in—an employment program for the handicapped which has proven to be highly successful.

Another question which frequently is raised in employment interviews concerns the firing or dismissal of the employee and the employer's reluctance to treat the rehabilitant in the same manner he would treat other employees. The counselor again will have to rely on his own resources; however, an analogy may be helpful here.

Indicate that if you, as a salesman, were selling refrigerators and the employer bought one which later malfunctioned, you would stand by your product and attempt to get it in good working order. The counselor could briefly discuss follow-up procedures with the employer at this time. He might also indicate that once the handicapped employee has worked for the employer for a time, the employer will feel that he is a fully functioning, well-adjusted employee who should be treated just as all other employees are. Assure the employer of your confidence in the client.

A fourth question which counselors must be ready to answer concerns architectural barriers and physical limitations of the work setting. Counselors should be frank in their responses to questions concerning limitations of the client and restrictions imposed by the work setting. The counselor should be the first to indicate that certain jobs are infeasible for many of his clients. He should be certain to get across to the employer that he is not going to place a client on an unsafe job or on a job which he cannot handle.

A fifth question which often arises concerning employment of the handicapped is that of the "second injury" which might result in total disability and effect the workman's compensation payments made by the employer. In a vast majority of states and the District of Columbia and Puerto Rico, "second injury" funds or equivalent arrangements have been established. In these localities, the employer is responsible only for the last injury and the employee is conpensated for the disability which results from combined injuries.

SOME GUIDELINES AND TOOLS IN LOCATING EMPLOYMENT OPPORTUNITIES

1. The counselor should be aware of industrial developments within the area that he serves and in adjacent areas.
2. The three volumes of the *Dictionary of Occupational Titles* (1965) offer a wealth of useful information for rehabilitation staff and facilities. Much emphasis is given to descriptions of physical and personality requirements for various jobs. In addition, these volumes can help expand the counselor's concepts about various types of jobs which are related to the general interest area of the rehabilitation client.
3. Employers with whom former clients have been placed can be important sources of information.
4. Previously rehabilitated clients can offer many sound ideas about existing employment opportunities.
5. Local Chambers of Commerce usually provide an industrial index which lists types of work available in most communities. Counselors also should coordinate their efforts with those of the state employment service since the mutual sharing of job information can be valuable to both employment service counselors and rehabilitation counselors.
6. When placing persons on jobs in rural areas, the worker should consider enlisting the support of local community leaders such as doctors, city councilmen, postmasters, and religious leaders as well as Rotary, Kiwanis, Ruritan and other civic groups.
7. If the counselor is interested in assisting individuals in becoming small business managers and operators, he should get in touch with the Small Business Administration office serving his local area.

PROFESSIONAL PLACEMENT

In rehabilitation jargon, "professional placement" generally means developing client employment opportunities which require at least a college education. Bauman and Yoder offer excellent coverage of this area of placement as it pertains to work for the blind. Professional placement is "facilitative" work for the counselor. The counselor can help his client in terms of giving advice and information; however, he must be certain not to take the place of the client in securing actual jobs. The client must be ready to meet without the counselor with the employer to discuss his professional qualifications for work. When he has a particular problem, the counselor should be able to assist him with information which could be helpful during the employer interview. For example, he should be coached on how to present himself most favorably. The counselor might help his client develop a résumé or portfolio which would outline his training and give examples of any previous work done in the job field in which he wants employment. Other procedures usually followed in placement may or may not be appropriate according to the judgment of the counselor.

A worker in charge of professional placement may want to organize precollege orientation groups for clients. It will be necessary also for the counselor who is dealing with persons in training to inform them about services available while they are in training and away from their home area. If, for instance, clients are attending college, the rehabilitation staff and facility should help them become acquainted with college counseling center services at the institution they attend.

Effective professional placement requires long-range planning on the part of both counselor and client. Two years before placement (in training cases) is not too early for the client to begin planning with his counselor in order to solve problems related to his securing the type of employment he wants. The counselor will need to prepare by knowing who the prospective employers are and the requirements of the job.

GETTING THE CLIENT READY FOR EMPLOYMENT

Planning for placement does not begin once the client has had vocational training and is ready "skill wise" for employment, but when the counselor first reads the client's rehabilitation referral form. The rehabilitation worker must constantly learn about his client in order to effectively help him secure the type of employment he needs. Jeffrey has developed a job readiness test which helps in the evaluation of job preparedness of clients. While the total instrument is not applicable to all rehabilitation clients, certain questions are quite helpful with most rehabilitation clients.

Role playing is an excellent method to use in preparing a client for employment interviews. After going through a mock interview which includes a variety of questions, the counselor can give suggestions concerning how the client might improve the impression he makes with the employer. In role playing, it is helpful for the counselor as well as the client to play the role of the employer. Once this is tried, counselors will immediately realize the usefulness of this procedure. The client should realize that getting a job is not an easy task and that he, to the best of his ability, should participate in the job-securing aspects of placement. In some cases, it is an indicator of effective rehabilitation procedures when the client is able to, in fact, "get his own job," assuming of course that he is ready for employment. The ability with which the client will be able to do this will vary with his motivation and the severity of his social, mental or physical handicap.

The rehabilitation staff and facility must stress "training" as a partial answer to many of the problems of the handicapped worker. Overtraining a worker for a job which will affect his personal and family adjustment for many years to come is seldom done. In each case, the counselor must take an individual approach to helping his client. In the case of those who are educationally or socially retarded, various remedial programs may be necessary before actual work training programs can begin. In each case, the counselor must exercise considerable judgment concerning what his client needs in order to be totally ready for employment.

On-the-job training can be a very effective arrangement for client training. In many of these cases, the state rehabilitation agency will make "tuition" payments to the employer-trainer in order that the rehabilitation staff and facility may get the employer interested in training a client and evaluating his work. It may be necessary for the counselor to help the employer arrange the appropriate payment schedule for the client since he is not a trained employee and would not receive an amount equal to a regularly salaried employee.

Bridges offered four major factors which are involved in successful employment of handicapped workers. These remain as highly important considerations for the counselor:

1. The worker should have the ability to accomplish the task efficiently—that is, to be able to meet the physical demands of the job.
2. The worker should not be a hazard to himself.
3. The worker must not jeopardize the safety of others.
4. The job should not aggravate the disability or handicap of the worker.

Eight Common Misconceptions About Vocational Placement

1. Because placement occurs toward the end of the rehabilitation process, the counselor's responsibility to the client diminishes.
2. Placement is an activity which requires no counselor training and is a matter of matching an available client with an available job.
3. Client location of his job or "self-placement" cannot be effective rehabilitation work.
4. When a client is ready for vocational placement, the information in his case folder is no longer of value to his counselor since the client has been, in a sense, readied for employment.
5. Follow-up after placement always can be handled easily by phone or mail communications with the employer or client.
6. Labor market trends and job information and analysis are the responsibilities of placement specialists and employment service counselors, not of general rehabilitation counselors.
7. An employer will notify the counselor and the rehabilitation agency when he is dissatisfied with a client placement.
8. An employer will automatically call upon the rehabilitation agency to furnish him with additional employees when he needs them.

Rehabilitation staff and facility should be certain that their clients understand that it is not necessarily bad to be turned down for a job. Counselors should understand that experience has shown that nine or ten employer contacts often must be made before the counselor makes a placement.

Job Analysis

Every rehabilitation staff and facility should be thoroughly familiar with the techniques of job analysis for use in selective placement. The rehabilitation staff and facility has to be able to match the prospective worker's social, mental and physical qualifications with requirements of the job. Factors such as judgment, initiative, alertness and general health and capability must always be taken into consideration as well as the individual's social and economic background.

Job analysis should answer certain questions concerning the job. *What* does the worker do in terms of physical and mental effort that go into the work situation? How is the work done? In other words, does this job involve the use of equipment and mathematics, or does it require travel. Why does the worker perform the job? This component of the job analysis answers the question concerning the overall purpose or the sum total of the task and is the reason for doing the job. The worker also should understand the relationship of his task to other tasks that make up the total job.

Generally, the rehabilitation staff and facility should attempt to place clients on jobs which they can "handle" and which do not require modification. In some cases, however, minor modifications can be made with little or no re-engineering effort. The counselor will have to be careful in suggesting re-engineering of a job, since this can be a costly undertaking in many instances. The major objective should be that of helping handicapped workers integrate effectively into the total work force without major modification or change in the work situation.

The following outline can be used in evaluating a job which is to be performed by a handicapped worker:

   A. Name Used for Position Surveyed
      1. D. O. T. Title
      2. Alternate titles
      3. D. O. T. definitions
   B. Usual Operator
      1. Sex
      2. General characteristics

    C. Physical and Psychological Demands
        1. Activities
        2. Working conditions
        3. Skill required
        4. Intelligence
        5. Temperament
        6. Other
    D. Description of Physical Activities
    E. Description of Working Conditions
    F. Description of Hazards
    G. Steps Required to Accomplish the Goal of the Work
    H. Equipment Found in the Particular Plant Surveyed
        1. Identification
        2. Set-up and maintenance
        3. Modification (if required for the handicapped)
     I. Equipment Variations Which May Be Found In Other Plants
    J. Pre-employment Training Required
    K. Training Procedure
    L. Production
        1. Full Production definition
        2. Time to reach normal efficiency
   M. Interrelation with Preceding and Succeeding Jobs

RELATING PSYCHOLOGICAL DATA TO JOB ANALYSIS INFORMATION IN VOCATIONAL PLACEMENT

As a first step in getting to know clients well, the counselor should make arrangements to secure appropriate psychological information about them. He should either complete job analyses or use available job evaluation data to make decisions about types of information which will be of value to his clients in the job selection and placement procedure. In many instances, however, the counselor fails to synthesize information obtained from two of his most important sources: the psychological evaluation and the job analysis.

The counselor should take five basic steps, as described by Hardy, in developing a successful procedure for interrelating and using important information. He should:

1. Study the needs of the client and the types of satisfaction meaningful to him.
2. Make certain that valid psychological and job analysis data have been gathered.

3. Review the requirements of the job and evaluate the individual traits needed to meet job requirements.
4. Consider the environmental pressures with which the individual must interact.
5. Discuss the job analysis and psychological evaluation with the client so that he will understand what the work will require of him and what it will offer.

Both client and counselor need to have an understanding of the job requirements in order to make realistic decisions. One important move should be structuring a set of goals—a guide to help the client avoid useless floundering that gets him nowhere. What satisfactions is he seeking? What is important to him in the long run and what types of work or work settings will provide these satisfactions? These are questions which the counselor must help the client answer.

Maslow has suggested a hierarchy of the individual needs which the counselor must understand in order to evaluate a client's psychological status—his satisfactions and frustrations. In the usual order of prepotency these needs are for (a) psychological satisfaction; (b) safety; (c) belongingness and love; (d) importance, respect, self-esteem and independence; (e) information; (f) understanding; (g) beauty; and (h) self-actualization.

In our society, there is no single situation which is potentially more capable of giving satisfaction at all levels of these needs as a person's work, and it is the responsibility of the counselor to help his client plan for future happiness through adjustment on the job. The worker needs to help the client become fully aware of the social pressures of the job because these are as important to the individual as the actual job pressures. A client's ability to the social interactions of the work environment will directly affect his job performance.

The counselor always must ask himself what the requirements of the job are. This question can be answered superficially or in considerable detail. A lay job analysis can give superficial requirements, but the responsibility for an in-depth job description belongs to the expert—the counselor who will often have to give direct advice to the client.

Effective placement requires effective planning. Planning

cannot be really useful unless appropriate information has been obtained, interrelated and skillfully utilized so that the client and the counselor have a clear understanding of possible problems and possible solutions.

Follow-Up After Placement

A rehabilitation staff and facility often is tempted to consider his job completed when the client is placed on a job which appears suitable for him; however, the phase of rehabilitation which begins immediately after the person has been placed in employment is one of the most complex. Follow-up involves the counselor's ability to work as a middleman between employer and client in order to help the client solve problems related to his handicap which may arise after being hired. The counselor must be diplomatic and resourceful in maintaining the employer's confidence in his client's ability to do the job. At the same time, he must let the client know that he has full faith in him. The counselor, however, must somehow evaluate how his client is performing on the job and make certain that he is available to help if problems arise which the client cannot solve.

In addition to the worker's service to the client during follow-up, this period can offer real public relations opportunities for the counselor, especially when the employer notes the interest with which the counselor "follows" his client. The frequency of follow-up varies according to the counselor's judgment of the client's job ability and adjustment.

Agency regulations usually require that a final follow-up be done after thirty days in order to make certain that placement is successful before a "case" can be closed as rehabilitated. Counselors should also consider follow-up periods of sixty to eighty days after placement. Again, this helps reassure the client of the interest of the agency and the counselor in his success and can be of value to the counselor in further developing employment opportunities for handicapped persons.

In follow-up after professional placement, however, the counselor must forget the sixty-to-ninety-day period which is usually adequate in the placement of clients in nonprofessional jobs. A longer period will be necessary and this period will vary with job complications and severity of the client's handicap. Bauman and Yoder have recommended six months to a year for follow-up for most cases of blind persons placed in professional work.

Counselors will probably wish to schedule specific days for follow-up in the field. Generally, the period of follow-up is a time when the counselor sees the efforts of the entire rehabilitation process coming to fruition. If the job has been well analyzed and the client well evaluated and placed, follow-up will be pleasurable experience for the counselor.

Summary

The rehabilitation facility's responsibility in vocational placement must not be underrated. The decisions made at this stage in the rehabilitation process not only affect the client's immediate feelings of satisfaction and achievement but also, of course, his long-term physical and mental health. The rehabilitation facility and its staff have a real responsibility to "ready" the client for employment by giving him the type of information that he needs about the job and about holding employment once it is achieved. Placement should be "client centered" with strong emphasis given to the client's opinions about work and how it will affect him and his family. Counselors must be ready to answer the questions that employers will ask about hiring handicapped persons and about the rehabilitation program. Vocational placement is high-level public relations work.

The counselor must be knowledgeable about job analysis and must interrelate all medical, psychological and social data with job analysis information in order to be successful in client-centered placement. Once a placement has been achieved, the counselor must "follow-up" the client in order to make certain that he is doing well on the job. The client should have an opportunity to evaluate his job and also the efforts of his counselor in helping him decide on and obtain the job. Effective placement requires effective planning and counselors must constantly evaluate their knowledge of the world of work and their ability to interrelate information in order to assure real placement success.

We feel the rehabilitation facility should have a keen concern for the placement of the client. All too often rehabilitation facilities view their role as providing only discrete short-ranged services for the client. They feel if the state rehabilitation agency is purchasing work adjustment they will be concerned only with the work adjustment of the client. If the agency is providing training they will be concerned only with providing a high-quality training for the client. We feel to be successful the rehabilitation facility has to be concerned not only for the specific services which are purchased for their clients but also have to be concerned for the total vocational adjustment of the client. We feel all who intervene in the rehabilitation process in behalf of the client should be concerned about the ultimate vocational objective of the client.

REFERENCES AND SELECTED READINGS

American Mutual Insurance Alliance: *Workers Worth Their Hire,* Chicago, Illinois.

Bauman, M.K. and Yoder, N.M.: *Placing the Blind and Visually Handicapped in Professional Occupations.* Washington, D. C., Office of Vocational Rehabilitation, Department of Health, Education and Welfare, 1962.

Bridges, C.C.: *Job Placement of the Physically Handicapped.* New York, McGraw-Hill, 1946.

Cull, J.G. and Hardy, R.E.: *Vocational Rehabilitation: Profession and Process,* Springfield, Ill. Charles C Thomas. 1972.

Department of Veterans' Benefits, Veterans' Administration: *They Return to Work,* Washington, D. C., U. S. Government Printing Office, 1963.

Hardy, R.E.: Counseling physically handicapped college students. *The New Outlook for the Blind,* 59, (5):182–183, 1965.

Hardy, R.E.: Relating psychological data to job analysis information in vocational counseling. *The New Outlook for the Blind,* 63 (7): 202–204, 1969.

International Society for the Welfare of Cripples: *Selective Placement of the Handicapped.* New York, 1955.

Jeffrey, David L.: *Pertinent Points on Placement,* Clearing House, Oklahoma State University, November, 1969.

Lofquist, L.H., and Davis, R.V.: *Adjustment to Work—A Psychological View of Man's Problems in Work-Oriented Society.* New York, Appleton-Century-Crofts, 1969.

McGowan, J.F., and Porter, T.L.: *An Introduction to the Vocational Rehabilitation Process.* Rehabilitation Services Administration, July, 1967.

McNamee, H.T., and Jeffrey, R.P.: *Service to the Handicapped 1960.* Phoenix, Arizona State Employment Service, 1960.

Maslow, A.H.: A theory of human motivation. *Psychology Review,* 50:370–396, 1954.

Office of Vocational Rehabilitation: *Training Personnel for the State Vocational Rehabilitation Programs—A Guide for Administrators.* Washington, D. C., U. S. Government Printing Office, 1957.

Sinick, D.: *Placement Training Handbook,* Washington, D. C., Office of Vocational Rehabilitation, 1962.

Stalnaker, W.O., Wright, K C., and Johnston, L.T.: *Small Business Enterprises in Vocational Rehabilitation.* Washington, D. C., U. S. Department of Health, Education and Welfare, Vocational Rehabilitation Administration, Rehabilitation Services Series No. 63–47, 1963.

Thomason, B., and Barrett, A.: *The Placement Process in Vocational Rehabilitation Counseling.* Washington, D. C., U. S. Department of Health, Education and Welfare, Office of Vocational Rehabilitation, GTP Bull. No. 2, Rehabilitation Service Series No. 545, 1960.

U. S. Employment Service: *Dictionary of Occupational Titles.* Washington, D. C., U. S. Government Printing Office, 1965.

U. S. Employment Service: *Selected Placement for the Handicapped* (Rev. Ed.). Washington, D. C.: U. S. Government Printing Office, 1945.

Weiss, D.J., Davis, R.V., Lofquist, L.H., and England, G.W.: *Minnesota Studies in Vocational Rehabilitation.* University of Minnesota. Industrial Relations Center.

INDEX

A

Abraham, Jacobs, 91
Administration, 133
Administrator, 119
Allan, W. S., 71
American Standards Association, 11
Architect, 5, 6, 7, 8, 11, 13
Asfahl, C. Ray, v, 14

B

Banister, Olive K., xi
Barrett, A., 215
Basically 4 Steps, 13
Bauman, M. K., 214
Bridges, C. C., 214
Brochures, 41

C

Carson, Gordon B., 36
Carter, Lowell, W., 84, 91
Case Recording System, 167
Cassell, John, 91
Civil Rights Act of 1964, 110
Client-Centered Placement, 198
Communicator, 132
Consultant, 118, 132
Consultation, 134, 162
    model, 65
Contract work, 37
Corwin, R. G., 147
Counseling program, 169
Cull, John G., ii, v, 53, 71, 162, 194, 195,
    196, 214

D

Davis, R. V., 215
DeJager, Harvey C., vi, 115, 118, 120,
    127

Design process, 7
DiMichael, G., 71
Dolnick, Michael M., vi, 37
Dubrow, Max, 91

E

Edgerton, Art, 84, 91
Entrance interviews, 105

F

Facility Development Process, 15
Fair Labor Standards Act of 1938, 31, 110
Fellows, J. Beverly, 84, 91
Flow Process Chart
    schematic, 18
    symbols, 17

G

Ganges, Arnold G., vi, 3
Gilbreth, Frank, 19
Gilbreth, Lillian, 19
Griggs, Robert J., 195

H

Halliday, Harry, 91
Hardy, Richard E., ii, vii, 53, 71, 162, 194,
    195, 196, 214
Human rights approach, 4

I

Information coordinator, 117
Initial training, 122
In-service training, 116

217

J

Jeffrey, David L., 214
Jeffrey, R. P., 215
Job analysis, 209
Johnston, L. T., 215

K

Katz, Israel, vii, 93
Kozoll, Charles E., 123, 127

L

Labor, Department of, 30
Lacks, P. B., 147
Learning centers, 115
Learning specialist, 117
Lerner, J., 71
Lesley, Philip, 92
Levin, Stanley, viii, 175, 195
Light assembly operations, 23
Lippitt, Gordon L., 116, 120, 128
Lofquist, L. H., 215
Loomis, Kathryn, viii, 72

M

Maslow, A. H., 215
McGowan, J. F., 215
McNamee, H. T., 215
Mulcahy, Frank W., 84, 91

N

Nadler, G., 19, 36
Nagi, S. Z., 147
National Labor Relations Act and the Labor-Management Relations Act, 111
Nolan, Nathan B., viii, xi, 148
Nussear, Helen, 84, 91

O

Obermann, C. Esco, 195
On-the-job, 124
Ongoing training, 123
Orientation, 122
Orzack, Louis H., 91

OSHA (Occupational Safety & Health Act), 111
O'Toole, R., 147

P

Paraprofessional, 121
Personnel Training, 122
　initial, 122
　ongoing, 123
　orientation, 122
Pfeifer, E. J., 68, 71
Planned Volunteer Program, 177, 185, 188, 193
Plax, K. A., 147
Porter, David B., 17
Porter, T. L., 215
Principles of Motion Economy, 19
Process layout, 24
Product layout, 24
Production Handbook, 17
Professional placement, 205
Program Accounting, 140
Program Planning and Design, 133, 136, 137
Psychological evaluation, 56, 57, 58
Psychological testing, 64
Public Law 91-566—Occupational Safety and Health Act of 1970, 36
Public Relations Person, 119
Public Relations Program, 72

R

Referral systems, 165, 166
Rehabilitation counselor, 54, 55
Rehabilitation Facilities, 129, 148, 151, 153
　definition of, 3
Research, 133
Roberts, A., 68, 71
Roberts, Rebel L., 92

S

Salmon, C. F., 21, 36
Salmon, F. Cuthbert, 21, 36
Sheltered Workshops, 100
Singberg, R. M., 68, 71

Sinick, D., 215
Site, 9
Speiser, Allen, 84, 91
Stalnaker, W. O., 215
State Rehabilitation Agencies, 158
Strict panel model, 65
Subprofessional, 121
Suchman, E., 147
Sugar Act of 1937, 110
Supervising psychologist model, 66

T

Terminal, 96
This, Leslie, E., 120, 128
Thomason, B., 215
Trela, James E., ix, 127, 128, 129, 147

U

Ulmer, Curtis, 123, 127

United States Department of Labor
Laws, 94
U. S. Employment Service, 215
Vocational evaluation, 169
Vocational Placement, 208
Vollmer, M. V., 147
Volunteers, 176, 177, 178, 179, 180, 183

W

Walsh-Healey Public Contract Act of
1936, 110
Weingold, Joseph T., 91
Weiss, D. J., 215
Work personality, 197
Workshop Director, 198
Wright, K. C., 71, 215

Y

Yoder, N. M., 214